LOVE
YOURSELF
WELL

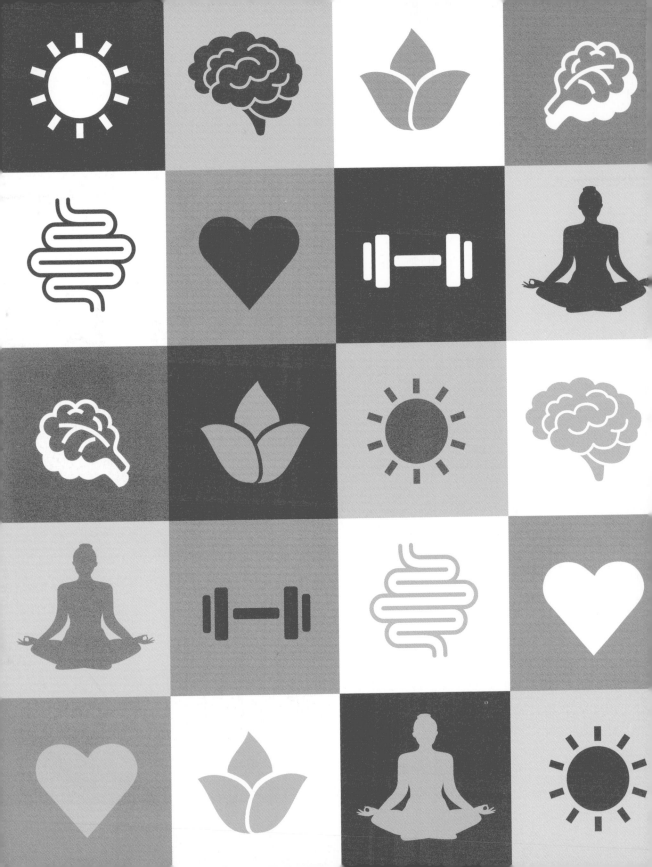

LOVE
YOURSELF
WELL

An Empowering Wellness Guide to Supporting Your
GUT, BRAIN & VAGINA

LO BOSWORTH

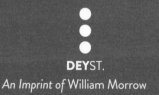

DEYST.
An Imprint of William Morrow

DEYST.

This book contains background information on different health and wellness steps, as well as the opinions of the author. The reader should evaluate all relevant information related to their personal health situation (not just limited to that which is in this book) and discuss all options with their medical care provider. This book should be used to supplement rather than replace the advice of your doctor or another trained health professional and is not a substitute for effective medical care or treatment. You should never delay consulting with your medical care provider or decline to follow their advice as a result of what you may have read in this book. The information in this book is not intended to diagnose, treat, cure, or prevent any disease or health condition. Every person's health situation is different, and no health and wellness plan will work the same for everyone. You should work with a trusted health care provider to find a health and wellness plan that works best for you, given your personal health considerations. If you know or suspect you have a health problem, it is recommended that you seek your physician's advice before embarking on any medical program or treatment. All efforts have been made to assure the accuracy of the information contained in this book as of the date of publication. This publisher and the author disclaim liability for any medical outcomes that may occur as a result of applying the methods suggested in this book.

HarperCollins books may be purchased for educational, business, or sales promotional use. For information, please email the Special Markets Department at SPsales@harpercollins.com.

FIRST EDITION

DESIGNED BY
Alison Bloomer

ICON IMAGES
© Shutterstock

Library of Congress Cataloging-in-Publication Data has been applied for.

ISBN 978-0-06-321789-8

22 23 24 25 26   WOR   10 9 8 7 6 5 4 3 2 1

FOR THE LOVE WELLNESS TEAM
PAST, PRESENT, AND FUTURE.
I AM NOTHING WITHOUT ALL OF YOU.

—LB

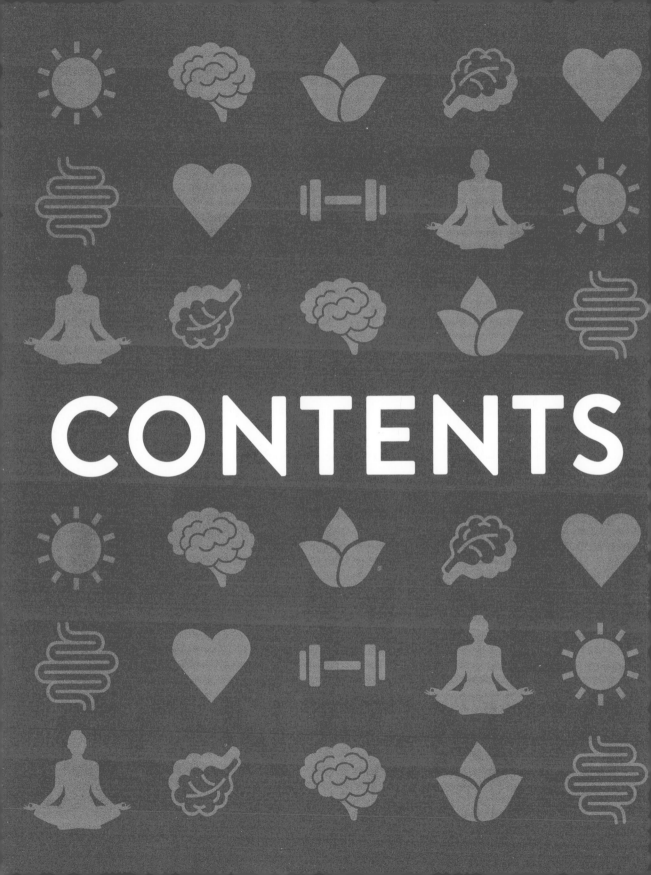

CONTENTS

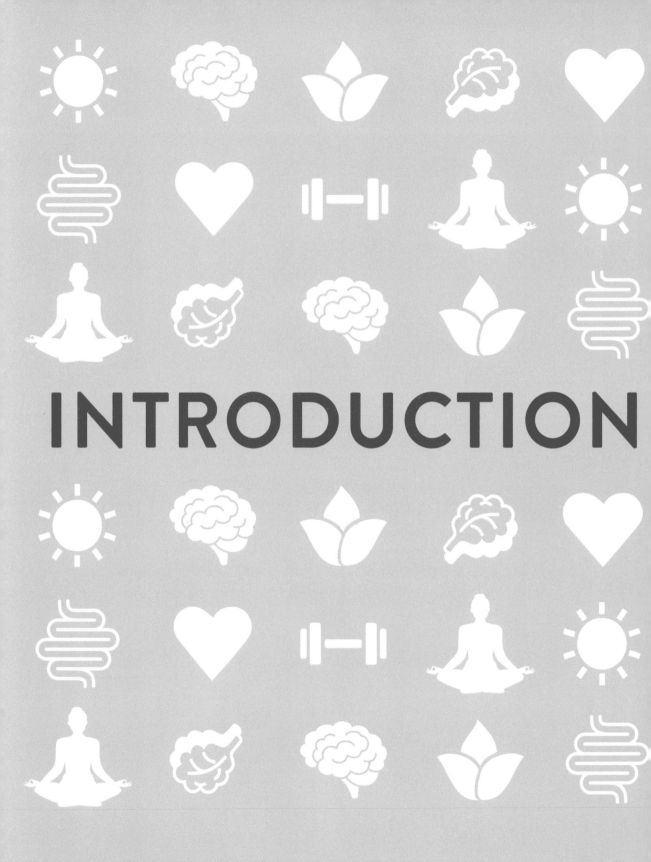

INTRODUCTION

Everything was going well for me in 2014. I was living in New York City, in a serious relationship, and working as a content creator in the lifestyle and food space. I wasn't completely sure about the direction of my career or how the relationship was going to play out, but I generally felt like life was unfolding for me in a good way. And then it all blew up.

One morning, I woke up and my heart was racing. I had an uncomfortable tingling sensation all over my body and a tightening in my throat that made it hard to breathe. I'd had similar episodes before, but never this intense or without warning. "Panic attack" is such an apt phrase. It felt like my body was under siege, and I remember in that moment I genuinely thought I was dying.

The panic attack faded after an hour, so I thought it was a weird one-off. If it was just a blip, I didn't need to freak out about it. But it happened again the next morning, and then the morning after that, and the morning after *that*. Soon, the panic attacks started to strike randomly throughout the day, too.

My life became divided into the time *before* that first morning panic attack, and *after*. *Before*, when I would get anxiety, I visualized the fretful feelings as water rising to the halfway mark in a glass. As I calmed down, the glass slowly drained of anxiety, until it was empty. *After* my morning attacks began, I visualized the anxiety as water filling the glass until it overflowed, poured down the sides, and flooded the room. There was no off switch for it. It just kept flowing.

I would drag myself through the workday and then collapse into the couch, too tired to do anything but zone out in front of the television or scroll on my phone. On a good night, I'd crawl into bed at 10:30 p.m. and wake up eleven hours later at 9:30 a.m. with a jolt of panic. I lost whole weekends in bed, finding it impossible to do anything else.

My boyfriend and I were at the critical stage in the relationship of looking at each other and wondering, *Are you the one?* Both of us were beginning to realize that the answer was probably "no." Our relationship hadn't been perfect for a while, but it must have been shocking for him to find his formerly upbeat girlfriend incapacitated by anxiety, lying on the couch, and sobbing for hours a day. (Not an exaggeration.)

Deep down, I suspected that something was seriously wrong with me on a physiological level. Why else would these attacks keep happening? It didn't make sense unless something was really wrong. But when I talked to my friends and parents about what I was going through, I got the kind of advice I might've given to a friend in my situation. It was the same advice I gave to myself: "You're upset about your relationship. Things are weird with work. *You need to meditate.*"

It's only human nature to grasp for easy explanations, and I *wanted* to blame emotional stress for what was happening to me. I convinced myself that my slowly unraveling relationship and the lifestyle of being a content creator were the causes of my anxiety. I was working as a freelancer and doing a lot of filming at home by myself, so it made sense that I was stressed in part because of the isolation that comes with the job.

I started seeing a psychologist who took my complaint at face value. She suggested that the tightening of my throat during the panic attacks was due to repression. "You feel literally choked up, like you're unable to say the things that you want in your relationship and in your life," she said. It sounded like an interesting insight, and when a therapist tells you something that seems to make sense, you internalize it. So when I woke up every day feeling unable to move, I thought, *I'm holding stuff in.*

Along with weekly therapy sessions, I was prescribed an antidepressant and Klonopin for anxiety. The psychologist didn't ask about my diet or sleep and exercise habits, though she did include occasional reminders to drink less alcohol.

I took the medication and poured my heart out in the sessions, but my anxiety wasn't getting any better. In fact, it was getting worse. I went to a cardio dance class, expecting to feel better, like I usually did after intense exercise. During the class, my levels of the stress hormones cortisol and adrenaline rose, a normal physiological response. Which would have been fine, except by then my mind was so conditioned to link those responses to the beginnings of panic attacks, so guess what happened? Well, I flew into one in the middle of the class, burst into tears, and ran out of there.

A few months into my health mystery, I started to get severe brain fog and dizzy spells. Not being able to think or speak clearly felt like being removed from the sharp, articulate person I had been. I remember once standing at the door of my apartment in Tribeca, trying to put my key in the lock, and the world suddenly tilted off its axis. I had to sit down with my back against the wall in the hallway for a few minutes before I could try to insert the key again.

This is not normal, I kept thinking. Why would an impending breakup cause dizziness and brain fog? It was getting harder to justify my symptoms as purely emotional. I was doing everything right and not getting any relief. Feeling helpless only added to my stress.

I pressed the issue with my primary care physician (PCP). She referred me to an ear-nose-throat (ENT) specialist who tested me for inner-ear conditions and suggested I cut down on salt. That didn't help. The spinning episodes came more frequently than ever and were chased by a fun new symptom, a constant ringing in my ears called tinnitus.

"The tinnitus might indicate an underlying problem," said my PCP.

"Like what?" I asked, desperate for any clue about my conditions.

"Well, I don't know," she said. "You have a handful of low-grade chronic mystery symptoms that don't point to a specific diagnosis. I see that fairly often, actually."

My primary care doctor might've thought that I'd take comfort in knowing that many of her patients had low-grade quality of life problems that weren't tied to a specific diagnosis or illness, but seeing the person I turned to for answers basically shrug off my symptoms had the opposite effect.

My psychologist told me not to underestimate the impact of depression. I wasn't underestimating *anything*. The majority opinion of my health care providers told me that my symptoms were emotionally based. So what was I supposed to do? Shrug off debilitating panic attacks, spinning head, and brain fog? I kept insisting, "There *has* to be something else going on." My physical discomfort was just too intense and worsening, despite medication and therapy.

As the months passed, I added new "low-grade chronic mystery symptoms" to the list, like urinary tract infections (UTIs), vaginal yeast infections, and bloating. For UTIs, I was prescribed antibiotics, often over the phone. For the yeast infections, I followed a frustrating pattern of going to the obstetrician/gynecologist (ob/gyn) and getting a prescription for Diflucan—the standard protocol. The itching, redness, and pain would clear up for two or three weeks, and then I'd get hit with a rebound infection. As for the bloating, my whole body felt puffy. I could press on my ankle and leave a fingertip-shaped depression in the skin. It was like pre-period water retention, but worse, because it was happening all month long.

By 2015, I was stuck in a revolving door of doctors' appointments and therapy sessions. Even though I wasn't seeing any positive results, I wasn't going to let go of these problems until I'd figured them out. So I followed my doctors' instructions to the letter and would then come back with more complaints. They kept writing prescriptions for pills and medications and blaming my depression. Admittedly, my emotional condition *was* terrible. Who wouldn't be depressed after a year of frustration?

"I don't think this is about my relationship winding down," I said on repeat. "I've been through breakups before, but they didn't cause bloating and yeast infections."

I was only trying to advocate for myself and get answers about my deteriorating health. When I pushed back—always politely—against the "It's all in your head" diagnosis, medical professionals doubled down on it. When I showed frustration, anger, and desperation—any emotions—it seemed to confirm to them that my symptoms were emotionally based.

Did they think I was a hypochondriac? A basket case? An attention seeker? Probably all of the above. I got the feeling doctors suppressed eye rolls when they saw me in their office, thinking, *Jeez, you again?* That didn't make it easier to advocate for myself, but I also knew I couldn't keep living the way I was—I was absolutely miserable.

A year and a half into my health mystery, my boyfriend and I decided to end our relationship. Although the breakup was coming for months, when it finally happened, I was totally heartbroken. I felt abandoned by him. We weren't married; we hadn't taken the vow of "in sickness and in health." I had no right to expect him to stay with me because I was ill. But I needed support, and I didn't have it from him any longer.

Ironically, the breakup and a breakthrough happened around the same time.

At yet another office visit, my PCP said, "Let's do a blood panel and check your vitamin levels."

"Okay," I said. It seemed like something she ought to have done eighteen months ago. I rolled up my sleeve and gave a couple of vials of blood. Drained, I went back home and got in bed.

Two days later, I received an email from my doctor that said, "Lauren, what you've been saying makes total sense now. Your vitamin B and D levels are severely deficient. It needs to be addressed immediately. Come to the office ASAP so that we can work on this."

I burst into tears. The relief was overwhelming. Finally, we had evidence that something was truly wrong with me on a physical level.

I called my parents and read them the email while sobbing. "I *knew* it," I kept saying. I'd been told that I was mistaken for so long, being proven right was hugely validating. It felt like a hard-won battle. Despite my therapist's theory that I'd been repressing my voice, I *had* been speaking up. The problem was that no one had been listening.

In the email, my PCP had attached the lab report. My vitamin levels were *all* out of whack, but the B and D levels were shockingly out of normal range. Within seconds, I started googling, and it was all there. Vitamin D and B deficiencies cause neurological symptoms, depression, anxiety, fatigue, dizziness, brain fog, much of what I'd been experiencing. I scrolled and clicked for hours, and I kept saying to myself, "Oh. My. God."

The next day, I went back to the doctor's office and received an injection of vitamin B12 on the spot. My course of treatment would be to get another B12 shot weekly for a year and then monthly for another year. A vitamin D deficiency is quite common, I learned. Humans absorb vitamin D through the skin from exposure to the sun. For more than a year, I hadn't gone outside much, due to depression, sleeping all weekend, and not having an office job to commute to. I started taking 5000 IUs of vitamin D3 orally per day.

Once we'd found the first clue about why I had all those mystery symptoms, we found others. More testing revealed a genetic predisposition that makes it harder for me to absorb nutrients, including vitamins and minerals that boost the immune system. No wonder I was getting chronic infections. As a kid, I would come down with one terrible bout after another: bronchitis, UTIs, ear infections. Every winter, without fail, I got the flu. Now I could see that I was prone to vitamin deficiency and infection. The warning signs had always been there, they'd just gone unnoticed. As my doctor explained, I could have had hours of sun exposure a day and eaten nothing but D-fortified and B12-rich food, and it still wouldn't have been enough for me. The doctors recommended supplements.

Until then, I'd always thought, *I don't need that stuff.* I ate fruits and vegetables and believed that I could get all the nutrients I needed from food. Turned out that was not the case for me. Nine out of ten Americans have a vitamin deficiency[1] and are probably not aware of it. Doctors don't often suggest getting vitamin levels tested, and those tests might not be covered by insurance (though at least they're inexpensive!).

The good news is that after a few months of B12 injections and D3 pills, I felt my exhaustion and brain fog begin to resolve. My feelings of depression and anxiety lessened. I had a lot more energy and a general feeling of improved health and wellness. Still, the supplements weren't magic bullets. It would be another year before my levels stabilized and I felt back to normal as I remembered it.

The very bad news was that my yeast infections would not quit. Since pushing my primary care doctor led to the bloodwork that revealed so much, I pushed my ob/gyn harder for answers. When she hit an ideas wall, I went to a new doctor. When that doctor came up empty, I found another. My *fourth* ob/gyn listened to my story and casually asked, "Have you ever heard of boric acid?"

"No, what's that?" I asked.

"It's an old school approach," she said. "A lot of my patients experiencing similar issues try boric acid if antifungals [like Diflucan] and antibiotics don't work. It can be life changing for them."

I said, "I'm down for anything."

"Boric acid comes in suppository form, but you can't just go buy a box at the drug store like Monistat. You have to get them custom made at a compounding pharmacy. It's expensive and it could take a couple days," she warned.

"No problem," I said. I was focused on the "life changing" part.

"I was wondering, have you taken a lot of antibiotics in your life?" she asked.

"Tons," I said.

"That could be one of the reasons why you keep getting these infections."

"*What?*"

Antibiotics could *cause* chronic infection? I'd taken antibiotics three times a year or more since childhood. This isn't uncommon for millennials. We are the Antibiotic Generation. Whenever we got a rash or had pain in our ears, our pediatricians wrote a prescription. Growing up, I would finish a vial of pills, feel better, get hit with a new infection a few months later, start a new prescription, and so on. It rolled like that for years. I'm not knocking antibiotics. They are miracle drugs, and we are lucky to have them. But what I've found out is that overuse and improper use of antibiotics can create resistance to them, and then it can become harder to fight off an infection. In that case, the more you take, the more you may need.

The ob/gyn added, "Along with the boric acid suppositories, why don't you try incorporating a probiotic into your daily routine? If you can find one made with bacterial strains that support women's health—there are one or two out there—that could also be really helpful."

Honestly, I wasn't quite sure what a probiotic was. As soon as I got home, I dove into a research rabbit hole and learned for the first time about the microbiome, the "world within" of trillions of cells of bacteria, yeast, and fungi that live in the digestive tract, urinary tract, female reproductive tract, nasal passages, and on our skin.

Taking antibiotics to kill the pathogenic (bad) bacteria that causes infection is a good thing. But antibiotics can also wipe out beneficial (good) bacteria that helps us. Killing our friends along with our enemies can potentially lead to another set of problems. For example, friendly bacteria in the gut aid in vitamin absorption and boost the immune system. If we annihilate gut probiotics (friendly bacteria), it might result in a vitamin deficiency. Good bacteria in the vagina maintain a healthy acidic pH level that prevents an overgrowth of yeast. If we kill off friendly vagina bacteria, it might lead to unnecessary vaginal odor or even an infection.

It blew my mind that a lifetime of taking antibiotics might be a contributing factor to my poor vitamin absorption and chronic yeast infections. Taking probiotic supplements—live strains of beneficial bacteria in capsules—could help maintain populations of good bacteria and support a healthy balance of the microbiomes in my gut and vagina (more about how this works later in the book!).

With a sudden, sickening flash of insight, I remembered that a few months before my first wake-up panic attack, a dermatologist prescribed me a daily antibiotic for acne. That prescription, I thought, must have been the tipping point. I was coming to realize that all of the things I'd done my whole life—all those things I thought were good for me—may have fixed problems in the moment, but they also seemed to have contributed to certain aspects of my health worsening over the years.

It wasn't like I could turn back time or untake a lifetime of antibiotics. All I could do was move forward. I was able to order a prescription for boric acid suppositories from a nearby compounding pharmacy. I was floored by how expensive they were as a custom-made product. As soon as I received the suppositories, I started using them. I also began taking a women's health probiotic daily.

Forty-eight hours later, I felt like me again.

For the first time in what felt like forever, I wasn't experiencing discomfort. This, too, made me sob with relief. (As you might have figured out by now, I'm not shy about crying.) Why didn't I know about boric acid before? Why didn't my *three* previous ob/gyns suggest it? If I hadn't lucked into going to that fourth doctor who casually mentioned this option, I would still be going from doctor to doctor. Her willingness to listen to me and think outside the box allowed me to support my vaginal health and start to feel like myself again. My story had a happy ending, but gosh, while I was dealing with doctor after doctor not listening, I was miserable.

It seemed impossible to me that you couldn't just order vaginal boric acid suppositories online. Despite countless searches, I could not find any suppliers on the Internet. However, I did come across some forums dedicated to women's health where women posted about making their own boric acid suppository at home. Apparently, I was not the only fan who didn't want to pay a fortune or wait to get them.

My inner women's health advocate perked up, and I ordered boric acid and gelatin capsules to whip up a batch of suppositories in my kitchen. When all my purchases arrived, I put on safety goggles, protective gloves, sterilized my counter, and made my own supply. They were just as good as the pricey ones I had purchased previously. But the DIY process was difficult and should only be done in a controlled and safe environment. I figured if I could buy online from a trusted provider, I would. Plus, maybe other women who were making their own boric acid suppositories felt the same way.

By then, nearly two years had passed since my health mystery began, and thanks to vitamin shots and supplements, boric acid suppositories and daily probiotics, I finally had the energy to focus on my career again. *I might be able to turn my new knowledge into a business*, I thought. It was something I was deeply passionate about—a business that could actually *help* other women support their health needs.

What would the business look like? Well, I knew whatever personal care items I made needed to be doctor-developed, safe, and clean. If my experience had taught me anything, it was that you need to know how things interact with the body. This information is often as important as the project.

Another thing that would be critical was making the products *affordable*. (I don't think I need to explain my reasoning there.)

But you don't go from "It's so crazy, it just might work!" to launching a company overnight. I began a period of intensive education into this consumer category and the existing research in the field of women's health. I sought out experts, doctors, and scientists who were up to date and knew their stuff, and endeavored to learn more. My questions were simple at first, such as:

"I know douching is bad, but *why* exactly?"

"I've been told not to use scented cleansers on my privates, but *why* exactly?"

"Why exactly" was my new catchphrase. In school, we were lucky to get an hour of sex ed. During that time, did anyone mention that scented intimate products could impact a healthy vaginal pH? No. I was coming to realize just how much critical information isn't really public—not in the way it needs to be, anyway.

Part of my research was to buy and try a huge range of personal care products. In that aisle of big chain drug stores, we're given many colorfully packaged options of awful. But you wouldn't guess that from the advertising! Those products—such as lubricants, cleansers, and tampons—contain chemicals that can disrupt vaginal pH and the vaginal microbiome, possibly leading to dryness, irritation, or even increasing the risk of infection. Over-the-counter yeast infection products have ingredients that can actually worsen irritation. But who would know that just by looking at the products?

I took every penny I had in savings from my reality TV days, partnered with a team of food scientists and medical advisors, and found manufacturers who believed in my vision of supporting women's health and wellness. We went into a small-scale production of a handful of products: boric acid suppositories, a women's health probiotic, an intimate cleanser, and pH balancing wipes.

I didn't have any money left for marketing, so I posted about the products on my social media accounts and did media interviews. My message to women was to be wary of the products they put on or in their bodies. Many of these products seemed to be made without taking a woman's biology into consideration. Other options existed, but doctors didn't seem to recommend them because (1) they didn't know about them, and (2) they weren't mainstream. As I learned, there *is* a woeful lack of research and funding for studies about women's health issues, dating back to the very beginnings of modern medicine. I couldn't change that, but I could call attention to the fact that options do exist and that women shouldn't lose hope. We can get off the roller coaster by trying something different. My own experience was proof of that.

Major media outlets started referring to me as the "Vagina Lady," and I was fine with that. In some ways, it was actually exciting. By calling me that, I felt even more drawn to the mission of helping women seek out answers that can help them to take control of their own health and wellness and ask the right questions of their medical care providers.

Plus, a huge obstacle to women's health is being too embarrassed to talk about what's going on in our bodies. There is a stigma about having or talking publicly about sexual and intimate health, for everyone. The social taboo begins in childhood for most of us when we are trained not to call attention to our "private" parts. If as adults we blush when we say "vagina," we might be too shy to take care of ourselves. I offer myself as an example of someone who isn't ashamed to talk about my private problems on big, public platforms.

My efforts to destigmatize the discussion about women's health care were often met with skepticism. I was often asked, "Who are *you* to create these products and tell women about intimate care?"

Exactly. Why was a former reality TV star doing this work? Because others *weren't* doing it, and someone had to. Who better than me to speak about my own trials to support my vaginal health? I had a platform to tell women what I'd learned while working alongside a team of female experts who provided excellent information and collaborated with me to create safe and effective products.

My message—that we don't have to suffer in silence and shame—resonated. Women bought the products. They told their friends and came back for more. My company went from being a modest operation with a few products in my living room to a best-selling total body care brand sold nationally at Target and Ulta Beauty, among other stores, within several years.

The most validating aspect of this success is that everything I experienced feels worth it. If I hadn't gone through what I did, I wouldn't have created a company and a community that helps women and normalizes the conversation around intimate health. If, ten years ago, a psychic had told me that I'd say "vagina" thirty times a day, I wouldn't have believed her. I couldn't have foreseen or planned any of this. Now I'm completely dedicated to my mission to provide women with the reasoning, science, and information to take control of their intimate health and to ask their medical providers the questions that need to be asked.

Ultimately, our health is up to us. We have to take control of our own wellness by being informed and pushing back if we feel dismissed. It is within our power to feel good. All we have to do is love ourselves well.

You might now be wondering, *Okay, but how exactly do I love myself well? What do I do?*

Answering the question, "How do I love myself well?" is the mission of this book.

On every page, you'll find information, insight, advice, and tons of practical, actionable steps that will make you sparkle from the inside out. I'll start by explaining how everything works, and then I'll teach you how to keep a balanced microbiome, support your brain health, and maintain a healthy gut and vagina. I'll explain how those three body parts work together for whole-body harmony. As you read and digest the concepts, keep in mind these three main principles for how to love yourself well. Each one transformed my life; taken together, they may do the same for you.

1. Listen to Your Body

Lasting health comes from recognizing what your body is trying to tell you. If it's saying, "I feel tired!" you can work with that. Start with that statement, and then you can connect the dots to fix it.

In my case, nearly a dozen doctors missed some of the major issues I was having. I know that each individual doctor was only doing what they thought was best, but I came to learn that, in mainstream medicine, doctors can travel in their own siloed lanes and understand only their own specialty to the exclusion of others. For example, a gynecologist may not link yeast infections to brain fog. They'll send you on your way with an antifungal and never consider your gut health. I went into office visits expecting doctors to connect all the dots, but part of being an advocate for yourself means being educated about how your body works, using that information to push for the care you deserve, and speaking to your doctors frankly about what is—and is not—working for you.

Since the day I read that "severely deficient" email from my primary care doctor, I doubled down on trusting my instincts, listening to my body, and working toward homeostasis, a blissful state of whole-body harmony when everything works like a well-oiled machine. As a result of being a strong advocate for myself, I now look out for myself. I eat better. I sleep better. I exercise and have more energy than ever. I focus on wellness. Good health is beautiful, and I like what I see in the mirror (nearly) every day. I'm living a completely different reality now than I was in 2014 when I feared that I'd never feel good in my body and mind again. We can all have that confidence if we learn to listen to our bodies and stand strong in demanding more for ourselves.

2. It's All Connected

The gut, brain, and vagina are linked. The health of one depends on the health of the others. I call this the gut-brain-vagina (GBV) axis. If one part is "leaky"—not functioning as it's supposed to and even sometimes allowing toxins and disruptive substances to either exit or enter its protective border walls—the other parts can be leaky, too. This is what happened to me. I'll explain how each of these leaks occurs in messy and exquisite detail in the upcoming chapters.

As soon as I learned about the GBV axis, I became obsessed with it. I had no idea that the gut microbiome issues could be linked to brain health, and how an imbalance in one can potentially impact the other. Virtually nothing is out there in popular media about the gut-vagina connection and how leaks in the gut trickle down to cause deterioration in vaginal health. The GBV axis isn't widely known, but I have found ample evidence that it exists and that it is the key to achieving homeostasis. When you align your GBV axis and see how you feel, you'll become obsessed with it, too.

3. You Have to Make an Effort

When you don't focus on wellness and your physical health is spiraling down, nothing much else matters; not your career, your love life, or your bank account. All you want is to feel better, and if that doesn't happen, you feel trapped.

What stops you from loving yourself well? Ignoring the inconvenient truth about women's health: You can't take it for granted. You have to go out of your way to be good to your good bacteria so that it will be good to you. You have to support the GBV axis with intention, so it'll support you.

As a city person who cringes whenever I hear hippie talk, I say with a straight face that Mother Earth has given us all we need to be well. If we open our eyes to what we intuitively know is good for us—food that looks pretty much the same on the plate as it did when it came out of the ground, sunshine, fresh air, movement, breath, pure water—and stop doing the "easy" things like ordering takeout, living on our phones, and buying cheap highly processed products that are full of chemicals and toxins at your corner drugstore, we can love ourselves well and feel so much better. Remember: Just because something is accessible doesn't mean it's going to make your life and health better.

I'm not asking for anyone to be perfect—I mean, I may have two vodka martinis tonight. I eat cheese, and will take an antibiotic if I need it. But I am asking you to make more of an effort to love yourself well by doing the work of being informed and not making *too many* easy choices that may affect your health negatively.

I'm going to help you every step of the way as you make small-but-seismic changes. I have created a five-week program that will support your whole-body harmony. The key practices are to reduce intake of environmental and dietary toxins, make delicious nutrient-dense meals, take the Essential Five supplements that support the immune system and the microbiome, eat foods that feed your good bacteria, and adopt lifestyle strategies that neutralize the stress of modern life. Using my culinary school learnings, I've created twenty-four GBV axis and microbiome supporting recipes that you will love. I encourage you to discuss these steps with a health care provider who is supportive of your ongoing journey to improve your personal health and wellbeing.

I've been working hard to break the cycle of convenience that we've become so accustomed to as humans. We are so consumed by accessibility, ease of use, and the addictiveness of our screens that it has become hard to come back to our humanness and live in our bodies. I can't believe I'm going to say this, but to get to body balance, you might have to put down your phone, take a walk, or read a book, like, say, this one.

One more thing: This book is primarily about physiological health—the microbiome, immune system, the nervous system, the endocrine system. The bulk of the info within pertains to every human. If you have a gut and a brain—and I hope that you do—you will get valuable advice about how to improve the quality of your digesting and thinking. The vagina research and the gut-brain-vagina axis science pertains to anyone born with female reproductive parts and the issues that go along with them. Woman who does not have vaginas can skip those pages, or read them anyway because the functioning of the human body is just that cool.

PART 1

BODY BASICS

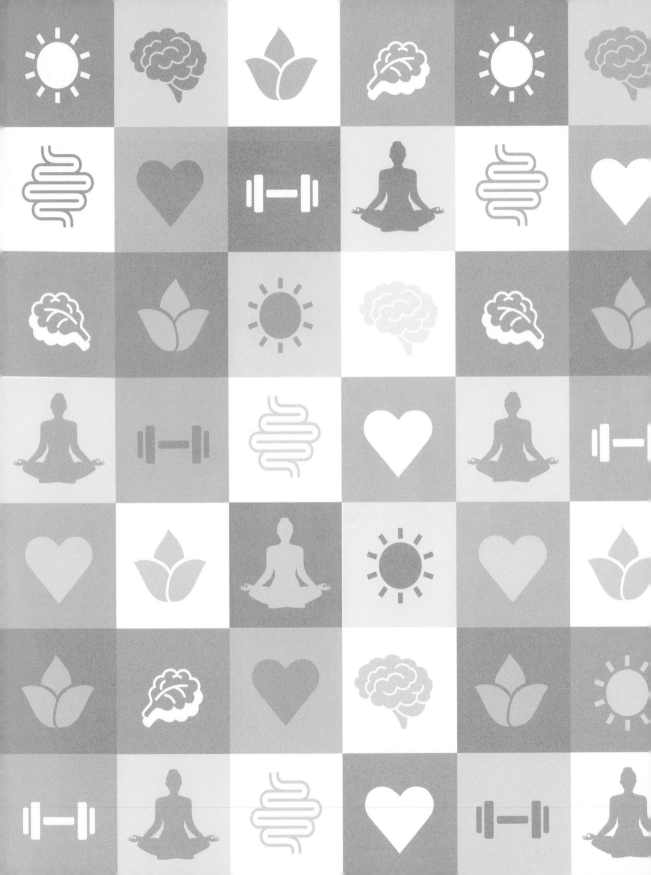

chapter 1

EMPOWERED SELF-ADVOCACY

"Hysteria" is defined as an over-the-top display of emotion by an unhinged individual or a crazed group of people in a "mass hysteria" situation. The etymological roots of the word come from *hystera*—Greek for uterus.

In the late nineteenth century, doctors and early psychiatrists like Sigmund Freud defined "female hysteria" as an illness caused by a malfunctioning uterus. If a woman was anxious, irritable, agitated, sexually forward, nervous, or had a tendency to cause trouble for others, she was thought to have a bad case of this dreadful condition. (Symptoms like fainting, shortness of breath, and loss of appetite were also attributed to hysteria, and not the far more obvious explanation that women wore lung- and stomach-crushing corsets at the time.) The treatment for hysteria? Marital sex, pregnancy, childbirth, rest, and "proximal convulsions," aka orgasms.

You might think this is an absurd footnote in medical history from a bygone era before we knew about germs or DNA, right? Sadly, no. Female hysteria was included in the *Diagnostic and Statistical Manual of Mental Disorders*,[1] the official guide used by psychiatrists in the United States until 1980, only six years before I was born. For women of my mother's generation, showing anger, sexual desire, or aggression would have been enough to diagnose them as unwell. It goes without saying that a man showing those behaviors would have been thought of as in the peak of health.

I bring up hysteria as an example of how women have historically struggled to get accurate information about their health. The brightest minds in the medical field once believed that the cure for a woman's disagreeableness was for a man to put a baby in her ASAP. I wonder how many women with legitimate health concerns were prescribed pregnancy by their doctors. No wonder they were angry and disagreeable!

"It's Hormonal"

All roads should not necessarily lead to your genitals. But in the medical community in the 21st century, women's complaints about their physical and mental health are often still attributed to hormones. I've heard about women going to their doctor to talk about burnout or depression only to be asked if they were on their periods. A wonky uterus is still the go-to explanation for whatever ails women. Jodie Horton, MD, an ob/gyn and a medical advisor for my company, Love Wellness, is often called to the emergency room at the hospital where she practices to consult with patients who have abdominal pain. "If the patient is female, I automatically get the call," she said. "I find myself asking the ER doctors, 'You do realize there are other organs in the abdomen that can cause pain besides the uterus, right?'"

Once, she was called to examine a patient who had been given a preliminary diagnosis of cervical motion tenderness by the (male) ER doctors. "After two minutes with the patient, I learned that she'd had a total hysterectomy years ago. She didn't even have a cervix," she said.

All the ER doctors had to do was ask the patient about her medical history. When the patient heard the doctors' cervical motion tenderness theory, she could have spoken up and said, "I don't think so!" But she didn't, and I understand why. Doctors present with a lot of authority, and it can be intimidating to disagree with them. Perhaps the patient didn't want to be rude and interrupt or embarrass the doctors for being so wrong. Whatever the reason, we need to get over that, because if we don't speak up for ourselves, who will?

A friend of mine was having intermittent pain in her upper abdomen, and her primary care physician sent her to get an ultrasound. When she arrived for the appointment, the technician informed her that a wand would be inserted into her vagina to check her ovaries for cysts. "The pain was under my ribs, not anywhere near my ovaries, so I was surprised when I was asked to take off my underwear," she said. "I immediately called my doctor and said, 'I don't need a vaginal probe.'"

After a slightly heated discussion, the doctor relented. The technician proceeded to screen my friend in the area where she felt pain and immediately discovered stones in her gallbladder. "I was glad to find out what was causing my pain and that I could schedule surgery," she said. "But I was furious that my doctor just assumed my ovaries were involved, and that I had to do battle when I was in that vulnerable position."

"Just Take an Advil"

On one hand, all female trouble is attributed to the uterus. On the other hand, legitimate complaints regarding a woman's reproductive tract symptoms are often downplayed.

I know from personal experience that an intimate health issue is always on one's mind. And if you do manage to forget about it for a minute, you're reminded as soon as you try to walk down the street. The thought of sexual activity while one has a vaginal infection can trigger shame, anxiety, and guilt, and partners are not always understanding and empathetic. Of course, you want the problem solved immediately. You want the pain to go away. Unfortunately, it's likely that your complaints will be downplayed or outright dismissed.

A friend of mine told her doctor for years that her period cramps were unbearable. And for years, he advised her to "take Advil and use a heating pad." Finally, she switched doctors and, through a long process of ruling out causes, she was diagnosed with endometriosis. She endured nearly a decade of pain because her original doctor seemed to believe that she was exaggerating it.

A close colleague of mine felt unusually bloated. "I would get uncomfortable from eating one-quarter of my dinner," she said. "My main doctor examined me but said it was probably nothing. I told him I was in pain and *begged* for tests. My sister had had a large cyst in her ovary, and I was afraid I did, too. But he said, 'Stop being so emotional' and that my pain couldn't be 'as bad as all that.' The bloating and pain got worse, to the point that I couldn't stand up straight. I went to the ER and sat there in agony for twelve hours, but because I wasn't bleeding, they wouldn't see me." The next day, her father, a retired physician, got her an appointment with a former colleague, who felt her abdomen and noticed the issue right away. Within a day, a Nerf football–sized cyst was removed from her ovary.

"It's All in Your Head"

Hypochondria is a mental disorder of being obsessively anxious about your health. Fortunately, I didn't run up against outright accusations of that during my many trips to see doctors. But my doctors did bring up the possibility that I had "psychosomatic" illnesses, meaning my physical symptoms were caused by emotional factors, like work stress or relationship issues. It's an all-too-common practice that a female patient gets a referral to see a psychologist when, despite visiting multiple doctors, nothing seems to help her—which is exactly what happened to me.

In the 1970s, the FDA barred women in their reproductive years from participating in drug trials or medical studies, often justifying it by saying it was to "protect" their theoretical, future children. Further justification for banning women was that their hormones would muddle the findings and make studies more expensive. Male-participants-only studies became the norm, and the assumption was writ large that if treatment and diagnostic tools worked for men, they were good enough for the little ladies, too.

Of course, that assumption ignores biology. Women have different hormones, different body parts, different reactions to medications. Science doesn't even know every way that female biology differs from male biology *because that hasn't been thoroughly studied.*

Diseases that affect women far more often than men—such as migraines, autoimmune conditions[2] like rheumatoid arthritis and multiple sclerosis, fibromyalgia, chronic fatigue, and Alzheimer's—are often underresearched and underdiagnosed. So-called male diseases like heart disease are well studied, but the research sometimes excludes how the disease affects women. A man with heart disease might present with chest pain, but a woman might present with jaw pain. Because doctors are often looking for classic (i.e., male) symptoms, they can misdiagnose female patients. One study found that it can take ten years for a woman to get a diagnosis of coronary heart disease.[3] Really, the one-size-fits-all approach usually fits white males. We are seeing more younger, female, BIPOC doctors who might be trying to change this paradigm, but they are often hampered by using the tools and models they learned from their medical school professors, who might not be as up to date as they could be. It might take a while before medicine catches up to the needs of female patients.

The Paradox of Convenience Care

Because doctors are under pressure to see as many patients as possible in a day, a typical exam might be only ten minutes, with the doctor staring at a computer screen for most of the time. Why bother calling it an examination? The appointment ends when the doctor gives you a prescription and a bill. Sometimes, convenience care (as I call it) works. The prescription resolves the issue. But sometimes, it doesn't.

A friend of mine knew that she was having UTI symptoms, based on previous experience. She told me, "I weighed my choices: begging unsuccessfully for a same-day appointment with my PCP; going to urgent care, waiting for a long time, and forking over the out-of-pocket co-pay; or just taking the antibiotics I happened to have in my medicine cabinet from an old prescription. I took the pills, obviously. My symptoms improved so I finished the bottle and felt smug about taking care of it by myself."

Two days later, her fire pee came back. She *ran* to urgent care and was put on a different antibiotic while her urine sample went to the lab. Several days after *that*, she got the results. "I had a bad bacterial infection, all right, but it was resistant to the first and second antibiotic I took to get rid of it," she said. "So, I went on a *third* antibiotic in as many weeks to treat the same UTI." As you know by now, antibiotics decimate not only bad bacteria, but can go after helpful bacteria. Her treatment likely made her vulnerable to leaky gut, leaky vagina, microbiome imbalance, potentially lowered immunity, and, ironically, a new UTI.

This scenario is all too common these days, with teledocs prescribing antibiotics based on a two-minute conversation or an email. They treat patients over the phone without seeing or testing them, based on self-reporting from patients. A lot of times, however, patients are wrong about what they think they have. It becomes a vicious cycle. If you don't go in person and drop off urine to be analyzed, doctors won't really know the specific bacteria that you're dealing with.

Convenience care—teledoc, urgent care, and five-minute PCP appointments—might seem like the right choice when you are pressed for time and can't spend half a day at the doctor's office. But in the long run, it might take more of your time and cause bigger problems. The system is to blame, not the patient. People are self-diagnosing based on their history and what they find on WebMD and Dr. Google. If your primary care doctor can't see you until next week and you have a stockpile of Zithromax Z-paks in your closet, of course, you're going to take them.

The Trouble with Research

Doctors complain about patient compliance (i.e., patients not doing what they're told). But doctors are people, too, and all people get complacent. Many health care providers will stick with what they know and may not be interested in deviating from what they were taught as standard care. If the FDA hasn't approved a drug, they don't want to know about it. The ancient symbol of medicine is the caduceus, two snakes entwined around a staff. At times, modern medicine's symbol could be the ouroboros, a snake eating its own tail. It's driven by existing research on drugs, which in many cases is conducted and funded by the pharmaceutical companies that then use their own studies to market their products directly to doctors, who then prescribe them to you.

I am not anti-medicine or anti-science. Prescription medicines are important to health when properly prescribed and used. But I also believe you can respect the conventional medical system while being aware of its limitations—and often those sadly have to do with women's health issues. If men tolerate a drug well, it might become widely available, even if women didn't participate in its testing. The consequences can be dire. According to a report[4] by the nonpartisan U.S. Government Accountability Office, 80% of the drugs taken off the market in recent years— for heart disease, diabetes, gastrointestinal (GI) issues, antihistamines, and appetite suppressants—caused terrible side effects in *female* users. A report published in *Nature* found that U.S. women were nearly twice as likely to have adverse drug reactions than men.[5] But times are changing, if at a glacial pace. Now pharmaceutical companies have to prove their products are safe for males and females, races, and ages. Since 2016, about half of the participants in clinical trials for new drugs are women.[6] Even female rats are being used more in scientific research. In the next ten or twenty years, we'll see fewer gender-related bad drug reactions as a result.

It would be a game changer if there was suddenly additional funding to study how we can help with women's intimate health care concerns. But in the meantime, the standard care remains dominant in the field.

Many holistic health care companies are making clean, safe products that are working well for women. But getting a new drug approved is insanely expensive and can take upwards of 15 years. The cost and time frame make it impossible for some holistic companies to get their products ratified under the current OTC and drug approval system. The lack of inclusion of certain products in double-blind randomized controlled trials with results published in peer-reviewed medical journals means that reported outcomes are often only anecdotal. "Where's the literature?" is the refrain. The rare doctor will say, "I'm not familiar with this, but let me look into it." That is the doctor you want; someone who isn't locked into the same old approach, no matter what. In my example, every previous doctor said that my infection *should* respond to Diflucan, despite ample evidence to the contrary. So we have to look elsewhere for empirical and anecdotal evidence. It exists, and it shouldn't be ignored.

Love Yourself Well by Being the Bad Patient

Being the "good patient" isn't helping us, and might actually be our undoing. Women don't always feel empowered to push back or speak up when doctors question us. Like me, they might even take pride in following doctor's orders to the letter, even if the instructions don't make them feel better.

In one study I read about 981 patients who went to the emergency room with severe stomach pain, the female patients were less likely to receive pain medication, despite having the same pain scores as men. Women who eventually got medication had to wait 33% longer for it than male patients.[7] Either there was a clear gender bias among the ER doctors who, unconsciously or not, assumed women were overstating their pain, or women were afraid to make demands because they didn't want to come off as pushy or troublesome.

Think of a doctor's visit as being on a reality show. You're not there to make friends. I'm not suggesting you should be impolite or disrespectful. Just focus on whether your medical professionals are really listening to you. The bad patient isn't combative. She's insistent in her own advocacy. And be sure to do some research *before* the appointment so that when you speak up for yourself, you have a good idea what you're talking about. Some guidelines:

- If you disagree with a doctor, it's okay to say so.

- If they seem offended, politely explain that you know your body better since you live in it.

- If a doctor refuses to run a test or give you the information you need, ask for a referral to a specialist.

- Keep a diary of your symptoms as evidence that you are serious about your health, and they should be, too.

- Come in with a list of questions, putting the most important on top, and insist that you get answers for all of them.

- Take notes during the appointment so you can refer to them later.

- If a doctor dismisses your complaints by saying, "It's hormonal," "It's all in your head," or "Just take an Advil," push back hard. It might be too confrontational to say, "Would you say that to a man?" Instead, you could say, "Excuse me, I don't feel like I'm being heard."

- If a doctor seems opposed to your questions, assert your rights by saying, "I'm only trying to get information from you so we can work together to find solutions."

- If a doctor continues to be dismissive or doesn't have time for you, you owe it to yourself to get a second, or third, or fourth opinion.

- Don't worry about hurting a doctor's feelings by seeking out other medical professionals. You deserve the best care you can find, and if a professional is not providing it, move on.

- When you do your research, be sure to use reliable sources.

Your Annual Wellness Exam

You should go see your doctor for an annual exam, rather than only in urgent situations. Pick a date, say the first day of your birthday month, and mark it on your calendar each year as Check-Up Day. Many insurance plans cover an annual exam with zero co-pay. It's worth it for peace of mind and to catch anything before it becomes a bigger deal. If I'd had my vitamin levels checked at my annual appointments, I could have avoided a lot of suffering.

At that annual wellness visit, double-check ahead of time with your primary care doctor about the tests and procedures you expect to receive. These could include:

- Blood pressure screening
- Diabetes screening
- Cholesterol screening
- A pelvic exam and Pap smear
- Sexually transmitted infections (STI) such as chlamydia, gonorrhea, herpes, HPV, and HIV testing
- A breast exam and, starting at forty, a mammogram
- Blood work that includes checking vitamin D and B levels
- A dermatological scan for suspicious marks and moles by a primary care doctor or, even better, a specialist

A DOCTOR'S PERSPECTIVE

I ASKED A DOCTOR FRIEND for his take on doctor-patient communication, and this is what he said:

We usually only have ten- to fifteen-minute slots per patient, so if I tried to get through an annual exam checklist, along with addressing every question the patient came in with in one visit, something important could get missed. So I ask patients to choose their top three questions and make a separate appointment to discuss another five or ten in depth. I understand that making and showing up for two separate appointments is a burden. It didn't mean I was trying to take advantage of them or rack up co-pays. It was just a strategy to provide quality care and information.

As for the closed-mindedness of some physicians, I do believe many of them may not be as receptive to new things as they could be. That's a shame. New discoveries are made all the time, and we need to keep up with them. If a patient came in with a study or an article from a reputable journal like *JAMA* or the *New York Times*, I would read it and do my own research. Very often, patients come in with random things they might've heard from an unreliable source, and that's not helpful for either of us.

EMPOWERED SELF-ADVOCACY

Here are some to-dos for championing yourself in a health care system with built-in obstacles for female patients:

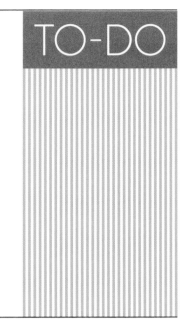

- If you have old pills laying around, don't take them. If your friend has old pills in the cabinet, don't take them. You know where I'm going with this: Don't take *any* expired pills.

- Even if you think you know what's wrong with you, get the lab work done anyway, just to be sure.

- Show up for yourself by going to the doctor as soon as symptoms appear. Take yourself and your problem as seriously as you want medical professionals to.

- It's more than okay to speak up on your own behalf.

chapter 2

LEAKY GUT

B efore anything else, maintaining a balanced gut microbiome and supporting digestive health is of the utmost importance. Vaginal health might feel even more important to your overall sense of wellness, but starting by establishing a healthy gut, with a thriving, balanced microbiome, is the key to the health of your *whole* body.

The Digestive System: A Quick Overview

"The body is like a doughnut and the entire digestive system is the hole," said Irwin Grosman, MD, a gastroenterologist at New York Presbyterian-Brooklyn Methodist Hospital. "Stretched out, the doughnut hole is like a long tube that runs through you. The tube itself is part of your body. But the space inside of the tube and everything in there is *not* part of you." Food that enters the mouth, goes down the esophagus, into the stomach, through the small intestine, into the colon and rectum, and out through the anus is *not you*; neither are the 100 trillion cells of bacteria, yeasts, fungi, and viruses that call the doughnut hole their home. "They're just along for the ride," said Dr. Grosman.

The gut microbiome (Greek for "small" and "life") is crowded and diverse. The entire human body has around 37 trillion cells; the gut microbiome has three times that number. We know of more than a thousand unique species that comprise the microbiome; science has only identified around 65% of them.[1] If you could scrape the microbiome out of your gut and put it on a bathroom scale, it would weigh three to five pounds.

As for how all these critters got in there in the first place, prepare to be amazed. When humans are born vaginally, they pick up their mother's bacteria from her gut and vagina. Breastfed babies pick up even more bacteria via their mothers' milk.

Children born by C-section and those who aren't breastfed start out with a deficit of gut bacteria, but they eventually accumulate them just by eating, drinking, and touching stuff. Every surface we come into contact with is crawling with bacteria, including our own skin (the skin has a microbiome, too; more on that later). We ingest microbes from hand to mouth, and then they move on to colonize the gut.

Hominids and gut microbes evolved together over hundreds of thousands of generations and millions of years.[2] But we've only been able to map the microbiome genome (every strand of its DNA) over the last couple of decades. Our understanding of how we and our bacterial friends interact is in its infancy. We do know that we have a mutually beneficial symbiotic relationship with them. We give them everything they need to survive: free food and a place to live rent free. In return, they help us digest, metabolize, heal, and function.

What constitutes an ideal microbiome? A dash of this fungus, and a pinch of that bacteria? Is there a combination of strains that will benefit us the most? "No one knows," said Dr. Grosman. "There are too many bacteria, yeasts, and fungi interacting with each other in ways we don't completely understand. You also have viruses that specifically infect bacteria and don't affect humans. We're talking about trillions of bacteria, which have billions of viruses. It's mind-bogglingly complex."

Because of this complexity, scientists haven't figured out yet what is good, what is *really* good, and what is not so good. Researchers are spending a lot of time, energy, and money trying to crack that mystery, and we might have answers in another twenty years. But right now, there is too much diversity in the microbiome—and too much variation from human to human, based on where we live and what we eat—for science to define a universally ideal microbiome profile for every person, racial group, or regional population.

Some of our gut bacteria are beneficial (good) and some are pathogenic (bad). "There is a wealth of research that proves good bacteria, also called probiotics, have a salutary effect on digestive processes and make you feel better. They can help us digest, absorb nutrients, detoxify chemicals, support immunity, regulate metabolism, improve elimination, decrease bloating, produce neurotransmitters and anti-inflammatory cells," said Dr. Grosman. *Lactobacilli*, for example, are readily available probiotics that can be found in yogurt, fermented foods, and certain supplements.

Bad bacteria strains can cause digestive problems. "A well-known pathogenic bacterium is *Clostridioides difficile*," said Dr. Grosman. "An infection of *C. difficile* can blossom into horrible, painful diarrhea, and it's very hard to get rid of." To kill it, or any pathogenic bacterial infection, doctors often prescribe antibiotics. Another treatment option is fecal transplant, whereby doctors introduce probiotic-rich stool from a donor into the patient with the gut infection via a minor surgical procedure or oral capsules.

(A side hustle you can really get behind, as it were, is being a fecal transplant donor. If your poop is well-formed—smooth, soft, solid, and shaped like a sausage or a snake—you can sell it to companies like Open-Biome for cash. According to the *Washington Post*, donors can rake in up to $13,000 a year.[3] Waste not!)

When we talk about beneficial and pathogenic bacteria, it's only natural to assume that we need less of the bad, and more of the good. But a healthy gut ecosystem thrives in balance. It's like how wolves in the forest keep the deer population in check, and vice versa. If one or the other population grows out of control, it can set off a chain reaction that throws the entire forest out of whack and can spell doom for the whole ecosystem.

The same delicate balance needs to be kept inside our guts. The best thing we can do for our microbiome balance is ensure that our probiotic populations are strong and not easily picked off by the bad strains. And one of the best ways to do that is to feed beneficial bacteria what they need to thrive: dietary fiber from plants.

What does all this have to do with a leaky gut?

I'm getting to that! There's just a bit more biology to cover first.

The Border Wall

Naturopath practitioner and Love Wellness consultant Gabrielle Francis, ND, describes the inner gut wall as your "inner skin." She says, "It starts in your mouth, runs through your entire digestive system, all the way down through the anus. You have an inner skin in the vagina and the nasal passages, too. The inner skin in your mouth is practically the same tissue as in your vagina."

The primary purpose of the gut's inner skin is nutrient absorption. Say you have a chicken Caesar salad for lunch. The salad enters the digestive system in the mouth, travels down the esophagus, into the stomach, then enters the small intestine where macronutrients—protein (chicken), fat (creamy dressing), and carbohydrates (croutons)—are broken down by enzymes into usable component parts, and absorbed into the gut wall. Protein is broken down into amino acids, fat into fatty acids, and carbs are turned into glucose or simple sugar.

The secondary purpose of the gut wall's inner skin is protection. Chemicals, viruses, germs, parasites, allergens like dust and pollen, and bits of undigested food are prevented from breaching the epithelial layer of the gut wall and passing into the bloodstream. A healthy epithelial layer has "tight junctions" that allow only the smallest of molecules, like water and nutrients, to get through. The microbiome's good bacteria live on top of the epithelial layer in the colon and fortify it, preventing harmful material from leaking through the gut wall and into the body. Germs, toxins, and allergens that stay inside the colon continue down that one-way street, out the anus, and into the toilet.

As stool travels through the colon, it sweeps up bacteria. "The percentage of bacteria in our feces is significant," said Dr. Grosman. "If you looked at your feces under a microscope, you'd see that as much as half of it is microbes." (Apologies in advance for any nightmares that image might produce.)

The third function of the border wall is to burn away infections. Your good bacteria play a major role here by helping to lower the pH level (toward acidic) inside the intestinal cavity (the doughnut hole).[4] When a germ or parasite enters your digestive system, it's bombarded by acidity that eradicates it, preventing it from sticking to the gut wall or migrating across it into the bloodstream.

In sum, a healthy gut wall or "inner skin" soaks up nutrients, keeps toxins from getting into the body, and burns off germs, all with the support of the microbiome.

Now We Get to Leaky Gut

If the microbiome is out of whack, with fewer populations of acidic bacteria burning off germs and fortifying the gut wall, your inner skin can become vulnerable. The epithelial layer's otherwise tight junctions can loosen and yawn wide enough for bigger molecules—toxins, allergens, germs, and undigested food particles (literal crap)—to pass into the bloodstream. The medical term for this phenomenon is "intestinal permeability" but it's known more widely as "leaky gut."

Some leaky gut complaints are:

- Frequent colds, flus, and bronchitis

- Worsening allergies and asthma

- Gas, bloating, constipation, diarrhea, nausea, irritable bowel syndrome (IBS), heartburn, acid reflux, and ulcers

- Rashes, eczema, acne, and psoriasis

- UTIs and kidney infections

- Yeast infections

- STIs

- Fatigue

- Brain fog and headaches

Leaky gut can exacerbate food allergies, sensitivity, and intolerance. If you have a food allergy, eating certain foods causes an immune response and severe symptoms like hives and swelling that may require immediate medical attention. A food sensitivity produces an adverse reaction that can take several hours or even days to show. A food intolerance means you have an enzyme deficiency (e.g., a lactase enzyme deficiency leads to a lactose intolerance) or a reaction to compounds in food (proteins in gluten, additives like sulfites, casein in dairy) that bring on gas, bloating, diarrhea, headaches, and stomach pain.

Dr. Francis, a practitioner of functional medicine that takes a holistic, preventative approach to find the root cause of disease, believes that up to 70% of Americans have some degree of leaky gut. Symptoms might seem innocuous at first, but if left untreated, they can snowball.

A twenty-eight-year-old friend of mine from New York said, "My symptoms started when I was eighteen. At first, I could write off chronic constipation as a lifestyle issue. I was a freshman in college existing on junk food. Things got progressively worse. By senior year, I'd either sit on the toilet forever with constipation or have to run to the bathroom with crazy diarrhea. I had terrible headaches, too, and took ibuprofen every day. The worst symptom was bloating with terrible, smelly gas. Once, in a crowded classroom, I was mortally embarrassed by it. I lived in fear of a repeat and stopped going to classes and parties. Eventually, I barely left my apartment." After graduation, she moved back home and was afraid to apply for jobs. After consulting with doctors, she realized she probably had leaky gut.

The condition isn't often diagnosed by practitioners in the medical establishment. "If you have tested negative for celiac disease, it's unlikely that a doctor will attribute your symptoms to intestinal permeability," said Dr. Grosman. "As we get better at measuring leaky gut in a generally accepted scientific way—which is starting to happen—the medical community will get on board with it as a disease in the larger population. Lack of studies doesn't mean it's not happening. But until those studies exist, we are very hesitant to say that non-celiac patients have leaky gut."

We do have research about factors that may loosen junctions in the epithelial wall to allow bad stuff to get into the body. The following list presents some examples:

- Alcohol
- Antibiotics[5]
- Artificial sweeteners
- Birth control pills
- Caffeine
- Environmental toxins
- Food additives
- Hormonal imbalance
- Nonsteroidal anti-inflammatory drugs (NSAIDs)[6]
- Pesticides
- Poor diet[8]
- Recreational drugs
- Stress[7]

Check, check, and check. The above might look like your shopping list for the weekend. Just being alive in the modern world and having fun can degrade the gut wall. "Everything I ate, drank, and took was bad for my gut," my friend said. "Once I knew what caused my problems, I vowed to cut out junk food, lattes, vodka tonics, NSAIDs, and then I'd be cured. Soon after this revelation, I got an office job and was extra motivated to be healthy and not have to run to the bathroom in the middle of a meeting. For two years, I ate perfectly . . . and my symptoms barely improved. It was disheartening, to say the least."

It doesn't matter if you're a vegan who only lets organic green juice pass between your lips. If the border wall has been leaky for a while and pathogens have been pouring across, you likely have another condition that is tough to beat: an overzealous immune response and the resulting inflammation.

Leaky Gut and the Immune Response

Our immune system is programmed to recognize what belongs in the body and what doesn't, what is *you* and what is *not you*. Macro- and micronutrients the body needs to survive are recognized as *you* by the immune system. When they pass through the gut wall, immunity central command gives the "all clear" and "stand down" signal to the frontline defense cells.

Foreign invaders like allergens, pesticides, and undigested food are *not you*, and if they get through the gut wall, the immune system alerts your body to launch an attack on them. This process is a beautiful thing. The body is doing what it was designed to do to protect itself.

The microbiome plays an important role in this process. Bacteria live on the gut wall, so they know before the frontline defenders—the 70–80% of our immune cells that live in and around the gut wall—if the border has been breached, and they raise the alarm to our immune system. A balanced microbiome signals an appropriate alarm. For example, if a small number of invaders breach the wall, the microbiome sounds just a few sirens. If the microbiome is imbalanced, the alarm system is out of whack, too. It might sound a five-alarm warning even if only a small attack would be enough to crush the invaders.[9]

An overzealous alarm throws open the immunity floodgates. The scorched-Earth, unleash-hell immunity response means the frontline defenders attack *everything*, including human cells they are supposed to be protecting. When those human cells are damaged, a new immunity alarm goes off, and more defenders rush in. The body winds up fighting a war to protect you, but the result can do you greater harm than the initial invasion.

Ironically, things we do to support our immune system—like hand washing and sanitizing—might make us more vulnerable to leaky gut. "If we're exposed to a lot of bacteria and germs in childhood, we have a greater tolerance to them and our immune system is less likely to react to them," explained Dr. Grosman. "If you were raised in a germ-free environment, and you went out into the world, your body's immune response would go wild. If you grew up with a lot of germs, your body will be more likely to shrug them off as no cause for alarm. Farm kids are exposed to more pathogens and are less prone to allergies. They build up a tolerance. In short, kids should eat dirt."

For a generation that grew up with bottles of Purell clipped to our backpacks and took antibiotics like Pez, it's too late to start eating mud pies now. Our tolerance for pathogens might be on the low side, but we can take steps to strengthen our border wall and balance our microbiome. It's our best strategy to a healthy gut.

I'll explain exactly how to do that later in the book, but first, I want to talk about how leaky gut can cause leaks in another vital organ: the brain.

LEAKY GUT

I'll go deep into how to help maintain a normal balance of the microbiome and tamp down inflammation later in the book. For now, here are a few strategies to consider to get you started:

- Help your good bacteria help you by eating more plants. Fiber is a probiotic superfood. The more you eat, the healthier your microbiome, and you, will be.

- Your bacteria populations do a great job of replenishing themselves, but you can take a probiotic supplement designed to support gut health as an insurance policy to help maintain balance.

- If you have any leaky gut symptoms, don't write them off as just lifestyle issues. Minor leaks from stress, eating junk food, and drinking too much can turn into bigger leaks, and then your symptoms could snowball. Talk to your doctor if they do.

- Gluten has been proven to activate zonulin, a protein that regulates the pores in the gut wall.[10] When zonulin is released, the junctions widen slightly, allowing bigger particles to get through, and signaling an overzealous immune response.[11] So start cutting down on gluten ASAP, and your border wall's pores will tighten back up.

TO-DO

LOVE YOURSELF WELL

chapter 3

LEAKY BRAIN

Leaky brain sounds like it belongs in a sci-fi movie with close-ups of gray matter oozing out of someone's ears. The condition is not quite so cinematic, but it can have dramatic effects on your mental and emotional health.
Leaky gut means toxins can get out of the gut. Leaky brain means harmful substances can get into the brain.

The brain does not have a microbiome (it's so sterile, you could eat off it—not that I'd recommend that), but it does have its own dedicated, amazing border wall called the blood-brain barrier (BBB). The BBB is composed of an intricate lattice fence of microscopic capillaries. For a visual of the BBB, picture the laser maze in a caper movie that surrounds a priceless treasure to prevent it from being stolen by Catherine Zeta Jones. In this metaphor, the treasure is your brain, the laser maze is the BBB, and the thieves are pathogens and inflammatory chemicals that want to steal your well-being.

Like the gut's border wall, the BBB isn't *completely* sealed off. Its capillaries are lined with epithelial cells that have very tight junctions and pores allowing only tiny molecules of oxygen and lipids (brain food) to get in, while blocking large molecules of toxins and allergens. Other larger molecules the brain needs—glucose and amino acids, for example—have to be ushered through the maze with the help of special transport proteins. ("Right this way, sugar.") Molecules of caffeine, alcohol, cocaine, antidepressants, and anti-anxiety medications are small enough to get through the BBB, which is why they're so effective. Many drugs prescribed for the treatment of brain tumors and neurological disorders, once broken down, are too big to get through the BBB, unfortunately, making it difficult to achieve good results. Drug makers are working to figure out how to make medication particles smaller or to sneak them across the BBB by other means.

If you are a healthy individual with a sealed gut, balanced microbiome, and an appropriate immune response, your BBB is probably functioning well as a fire wall to protect your brain. Good for you and your ability to win Wordle in three tries.

However, if you have a weak gut wall, an imbalanced microbiome, and an overzealous immune response, your BBB may be vulnerable. It can be weakened further by neurological diseases that trigger an exaggerated immune response.[1] But in the absence of multiple sclerosis, Alzheimer's, brain trauma, or cancer, I believe that leaky brain is likely related to leaky gut. Leaky brain has been linked to a microbiome imbalance,[2] which, in turn, causes leaky gut. It's no wonder that both leaks share many risk factors, like poor diet, infections, stress, environmental toxins, autoimmune diseases, and food intolerances.

How I believe that it likely happens: Foreign invaders enter the body due to gut leaks and are met by frontline defenders. But they don't necessarily stay in the place where they entered. The bloodstream is the body's superhighway that carries nutrients, oxygen, hormones, and blood to every cell and organ that needs them, which means it's also a convenient transport system for germs, viruses, toxins, and cytokines. If the BBB's tight junctions are battered by a torrent of cytokines, they can become "penetrant"[3] and allow big bad molecules to leak into the brain, with the potential to negatively impact mental and cognitive health.

The Damage

I don't mean to scare anyone, but the breakdown of the BBB has been associated with degenerative brain disorders, like multiple sclerosis, Alzheimer's, and Parkinson's disease.[4] Other associated issues can include memory loss, anxiety, depression, migraine,[5] and sleep issues.[6] Two leaky brain issues I endured were an impact on my cognitive health and mood. Some experts believe that chronic brain fog in one's youth may lead to dementia, Alzheimer's, and Parkinson's disease later in life.[7] It's fascinating to me how the antibiotic overuse that decimated my gut microbiome might have contributed to the effects on my mental health that hijacked my life for so long.

Leaky brain derailed my thirty-four-year-old friend's life for more than a year. At first, she blamed her symptoms on her demanding tech job that had her staring at her computer screen for sixteen hours a day. "I was taking four NSAIDs at a time for my migraines and a prescription sleeping pill every night for eight months. I knew it wasn't healthy, but I felt trapped. Pills were the way out," she said. "When it became impossible to concentrate for more than half an hour at a time, I thought, *I'm burned out.* I took an unpaid leave of absence from my job to rest. I felt less pressure, but I still felt exhausted all the time. My memory and focus didn't come back. I couldn't get through a TV show without losing the thread. When my leave ended after three months, I had rolling panic attacks about going back because I'd lost confidence in my ability to do the job. I'd always prided myself on intelligence. Feeling stupid was probably the most upsetting aspect of all of this for me."

As in her case, my mental health concerns could be explained by a syndrome I didn't know existed. Why would I know about leaky brain? Why would *anyone*? I hadn't read anything about it or its connection to leaky gut. It's not like the two organs are next door neighbors. I thought one was for digesting and the other for thinking. But the gut and the brain are connected, and when one isn't functioning well, neither is the other.

Because our medical system often treats the parts, rather than the person as a whole, many doctors aren't making the connection to how depression medication can make your symptoms worse. Not to say that you should stop taking medication. Just know that it's all connected.

Another leaky gut/leaky brain vicious cycle involves sleep. Poor sleep negatively impacts the diversity of the microbiome[8] and could lead to gut dysbiosis or imbalance. A symptom of an imbalanced gut is sleep disruption. Which came first, the imbalance or the sleeplessness? Either? Both? No one knows. It gets worse: Poor sleep quality plus gut imbalance has been associated with "low-grade inflammation" that batters the BBB and allows more pathogens and cytokines to get into the brain.[9] So sleeping badly and gut dysbiosis can impact brain health and further sleep problems that wreck the microbiome. It's a lose-lose-lose scenario.

You see what I mean? Once you get on the leaky gut/leaky brain two-way highway to hell, it's hard to get off because they make each other worse. In later chapters, I'll show you how to find the exit ramp.

If the effects of leaky gut can trickle upstream to the brain and cause leaking there, does it also trickle downstream and cause leaking in parts below the waist? Why, yes. Read all about it in the next chapter.

NEXT LEVEL BACTERIA: PSYCHOBIOTICS

SOME STRAINS OF GOOD BACTERIA in the gut have the specific job of supporting mental health.[10] They're called "psychobiotics," and might provide some help.

A study by researchers in the United Kingdom split its 124 female participants into two groups: (1) those that drank fermented milk with *Lactobacillus casei Shirota*, and (2) the control group that took a placebo. After the three-week study period, the participants in the fermented milk group who had initially rated themselves as having the lowest mood, self-reported to feeling significantly happier compared to their placebo-taking peers.[11]

In a French study, researchers gave fifty-five male and female participants either a probiotic mixture with *Lactobacillus helveticus* and *Bifidobacterium longum* or a placebo, for thirty days. Next, the participants self-reported on their mood. The probiotic group, compared to the placebo group, showed declines in negative mood. But the real proof was in the pee. Urine samples were collected before and after the study period, and the probiotic group's urine showed a decrease in cortisol, suggesting lower stress levels in the participants.[12]

A Dutch study used a similar format, giving participants either a mixture of several strains of *Bifidobacterium* and *Lactobacillus* or a placebo over a four-week period. The probiotic group had substantially reduced rumination tendencies compared to the control group.[13]

The best part? Taking probiotics for mood can also help support gut and brain health. That's a win-win.

LEAKY BRAIN

A healthy gut and balanced microbiome is crucial to cognitive and mental health. Here are a few recommendations to get that ball rolling:

- Eat plant fiber (aka prebiotics) as it produces the postbiotic butyrate, which can provide an all-purpose brain booster. Every time you have an apple or an artichoke, two key prebiotics, you may feel a little bit smarter.

- Cut back on gluten. Eating wheat, barley, and rye releases zonulin, a protein that, according to research from Harvard University, weakens the BBB's defenses, allowing inflammatory chemicals and toxins into the brain.[14]

- You're already taking a gut probiotic. In addition to that, take a daily psychobiotic supplement designed to support brain health and mood. Also remember to integrate probiotic rich food in your diet to help maintain a balanced mood.

TO-DO

chapter 4

LEAKY VAGINA

And now we come to the vagina, and the vagina-adjacent urinary tract. Although the vagina is the last GBV axis organ, it's number one on the list of Body Parts That Can Make Your Life Miserable.

If you have a leaky gut, you might feel off, with worsening symptoms over time. Same with leaky brain. But when the vagina (or urinary tract) is leaky, you will be painfully aware of it every second of the day. A friend of mine described the feeling as "like having a swarm of mosquitos buzzing around my thoughts." She said, "It was just annoying, but I couldn't stop thinking about it. I felt dirty. I obsessed over how it happened, when it was going to go away, how to avoid sex with my partner, which panties to wear, if anyone could tell I had it just by looking at me." Leaky vagina isn't just a physical condition; it's an emotional burden.

Knowing that your reproductive and urinary tracts connect with your gut and brain is perhaps the most important piece of the whole-body harmony puzzle, in my view. If I can get one message across to you, let it be this: If you have chronic leaks in *any* one of the GBV axis organs, you might be leaking in more than one place. You might go to a gynecologist for intimate health concerns, a gastroenterologist for tummy trouble, a therapist for your mood, and a neurologist for cognitive health. But all of these could be related to the balance of your microbiome and one or more organ leaks. Focusing on just one, under the care of a doctor who specializes in only a particular area of expertise, might not be a successful strategy for all. My intimate health concerns would ease up for a couple of weeks at a time, but they always came thundering back for a couple of reasons. I wasn't using the right medication. And I wasn't tending to my underlying condition—a microbiome imbalance that started in the gut and trickled down to the vagina, and gut leaks that could have contributed to the issue.

I'll bet you have never heard that the gut, brain, and vagina are connected—but they *are*, and it's amazing. In this chapter, I'm going to show you how.

Lady Parts: A Quick Overview

Our research at my company has informed us that between 45% and 50% of women can't identity their own body parts. Many refer to the entire female genitalia as "the vagina." That is not accurate. To take care of our intimates, we need to call them by their names.

The swell of flesh above the pubic bone is the pubic mound. The vulva refers to the external genitalia you can see with a hand mirror and good lighting, including the labia majora (outer lips), the labia minora (inner lips), the button or gland of the clitoris with its clitoral hood (the fold of skin on top of it), the urethra opening (the pee hole), the vaginal opening, and the perineum (the "taint," the region between the vaginal opening and the anus). The vagina refers to the internal elastic muscular canal that extends into the body and ends at the cervix, the hard, doughnut-shaped gateway to the uterus, the pear-shaped womb. Along with the vagina-cervix-uterus complex are the ovaries, oval egg sacs, and fallopian tubes, which catch released eggs and funnel them into the uterus.

The vaginal walls are porous, just like the gut wall and the blood-brain barrier. Unlike those organs (that everyone has), the vagina's permeability or leakability hasn't been researched nearly as well. We do know that small molecules of viruses, toxins, and medications can get across the border walls and into the bloodstream. We also know that the inner skin of the vagina is four times more absorbent than the outer skin.

When toxins get through the gut wall, the microbiome raises the alarm and an army of fighting cells rush to the site of the invasion and attack. When toxins get through the vaginal wall, the immunity response is more complicated. Compared to the gut, there are fewer immunity foot soldiers lined up for battle in and around the vaginal area. And the immunity army profile changes over the course of the month, over the span of a pregnancy, and over a lifetime of hormonal shifts.

The Vaginal Microbiome

The world within the vagina contains more than 100 strains of bacteria, yeasts, and fungi. Their main job is to keep the vagina pH acidic so harmful stuff is burned up before it can stick to the walls and cause an issue. They also help to block toxins and germs from crossing through the porous vaginal walls, getting into the bloodstream, and triggering an unwanted response.

The profile of the gut microbiome and the vaginal microbiome are not identical, but they are similar. Over time, the composition of each develops separately, but they often have many strains and species in common.

The gut and vagina microbiomes are in constant communication with each other, a phenomenon sometimes called "quorum sensing" or "bacterial cross-talk," where signaling chemicals allow bacteria in different locations to "talk" to each other about their environment, behavior, and population diversity.[1] Your gut and vagina microbiomes are kind of like tween BFFs texting back and forth all day long, encouraging each other's best and worst impulses. The gut microbiota can send a text to their counterparts in the vagina that says, "There's been a change up here. We need you to follow suit ASAP." And then the vagina bacteria will readjust accordingly and not necessarily for the host's (your) benefit.

The gut and vagina microbiomes communicate by another method that I call "bacterial cross-*walk*." The gut, vagina, and vulva are all lined with a viscous mucus layer. The gut's mucus coating ends at the anus, mere inches from the vaginal and urethral opening. Gut bacteria migrate from the anus across the mucus trail to visit, and influence, the microbiomes on the vulva, in the vagina, and in the urinary tract.

Whether these populations communicate via cross-talk or cross-walk (or both), the gut's probiotic breakdown will be reflected in the vagina as well. I call this phenomenon "trickle-down dysbiosis." An example: If there is an overgrowth of a pathogenic strain of yeast in the gut, it won't stay local. Unchecked, that overgrowth might become systemic, meaning it can spread to other microbiomes in the body that contain that particular strain. The vagina and gut share yeast strains, so an overgrowth in one has the potential to cause an issue in the other.

The Dominant Strain

You don't want a *basic* vagina. Everyone should actually think of their genitalia as *extra*—that's where all the fun is happening! Although in this case, the word basic is technically referring to alkalinity on the pH scale. A healthy vaginal pH is acidic, between 3.8 and 4.5 on the pH scale (the range accounts for individual variation). Ideally, your vagina is more acidic than black coffee, the same as red wine, and a little less than lemon juice. Even a slight shift toward alkalinity in the vagina can create a breeding ground for harmful bacteria and yeasts to overgrow.

A dominant probiotic strain in every woman's vagina is *lactobacillus*, which is working hard 24/7 to keep our vagina healthy. How? It produces lactic acid, which burns up germs that might otherwise clump on the wall and infect it. *Lactobacillus* also produces a substance called bacteriocin, the vagina's very own organic antibiotic, that inhibits the growth of bad bacteria and keeps the vagina in balance.[2] If *lactobacilli* levels are disrupted, yeasts (like *candida*) and bad bacteria that are already inside the vagina can take over.

Maintaining acid producing *lactobacilli* levels is key. What messes that up? Well, potentially, over time, antibiotics can disrupt them. When you take antibiotics for an inflamed cut on your finger, your vagina is probably the last thing on your mind. Think again. Wiping out *lactobacilli* creates a perfect environment in the vagina for yeast to take over. Antibiotics might make your finger feel better, and you can, once again, swipe left at a furious pace. However, with the depletion of good bacteria, your vagina could potentially be feeling the opposite. Of course, take antibiotics as needed! Just make sure to take a probiotic for women's health to keep your microbiome in fighting shape.

Leaky Vagina Nightmares

Some of the most common leaky vagina concerns are bacterial over-growth and yeast, my sworn enemy.

Bacteria overgrowth can be caused by having multiple (no judge-ment) or new sexual partners, douching (a product or process that is more harmful than helpful), and using scented soap. This may result in frothy discharge that might be green or gray, a fishy or a foul odor, and burning or irritation of the vaginal opening.

A happy vagina is crucial to your peace of mind, sex life, and physical well-being. Antibiotics, stress, uncontrolled diabetes, birth control pills, intrauterine devices (IUDs), and pregnancy are all risk factors that could upset that, and the microbiome balance in the gut and/or vagina is an important consideration.

A thirty-four-year-old friend of mine experienced recurring yeast overgrowth for years. "The part of my body that had brought me so much joy and pleasure in the past became a source of pain and stress. My stress and frustration were sky high. I just wanted a vagina that didn't seem to hate me," she said. "My boyfriend wanted my vagina not to hate him, too. It seemed like I was constantly waking up with irritation and redness. He felt awful about it, even though it was not his fault. Neither one of us knew why it kept happening. We would shower first, get clean, and practice safe sex, with condoms and lube. I started to believe that my anxiety about getting an infection was somehow causing them."

The tragedy is that sometimes the very things we do to keep our vagina healthy can actually do the exact opposite.

Things Not to Put in the Vagina

To keep a vagina healthy, you need to be painstakingly picky about *every-thing* that you put in and around it.

The many ob/gyn doctors I saw about my intimate health concerns warned me not to use scented soap. None of them explained to me why those products could be so harmful. Once I started doing the research for myself and my company by asking, "But *why* exactly?" on repeat, I got answers from teams of experts, who ultimately became my company's medical advisors. I think of them as the Intimate Avengers, saving the world one vagina at a time . . . including mine.

Bath soap is advertised as "pure," and can be *pure evil* for the vagina. It has a pH of 12, which is extremely alkaline—only a point away from bleach. When we wash our privates with soap, we effectively neutralize the acid we need to keep our vaginal microbiome balanced and ward off intruders.

As I'd been told to do, I used only water to clean inside the vagina. But I did buy a personal care cleanser at a drug store to use on my vulva. Sadly, if you use such products, as I did (as well as many others, with up to 95% of women potentially using at least one cleansing product there!), you're three times more likely to have vaginal health issues.[3] Many cleansers contain cheap chemicals and fragrances in their formulas. Even if you use them only on the vulva, they can kill beneficial bacteria there, before impacting your internal genitalia.

Many women do want to use more than just water on the vulva, and for that reason, you might consider using a safe and gentle cleanser that is doctor recommended and pH balanced. My advice is that whenever you shop for an intimate care product, read the label first. Some common ingredients in personal care products you might not know about:

- **SURFACTANTS,** such as sodium lauryl sulfate (SLS), sodium laureth ether sulfate (SLES), and polyethylene glycol (PEG). Surfactants are often put in shampoos, body washes, intimate, and face cleansers to wash away surface oils and dirt. However, they raise vulvovaginal pH[4], which dries out and irritates your tender skin, creating microtears where bad bacteria can harbor and grow. Lastly, they might trigger an allergic reaction and inflammation.

- PARABENS, such as methylparaben, ethylparaben, propylparaben, butylparaben, isobutylparaben, and isopropylparaben. Parabens are preservatives that make it possible for a product to sit on the drugstore shelf for dog years. Feminine washes with parabens can dry out and irritate your skin, increasing your risk of infection. Even worse, they can mimic estrogen in the body, which may cause hormonal imbalance, interfere with hormonal production, and impair reproductive functioning.[5]

- FRAGRANCES. Any product that smells like a walk in the woods or a rainy night in June might contain hundreds of chemicals (such as phthalates, styrene, and benzyl acetate). Some of those chemicals have been linked to conditions like cancer, neurological disorders, autoimmune problems, and central nervous system issues—and more. The FDA does not require fragrance chemicals to be listed on ingredient labels, so just to play it safe, it is recommended that you choose unscented products. Products that claim to have "essential oils" or "natural" fragrances can be risky, so you should be on the lookout for them, too.

Again, anything that raises your vulvovaginal pH can disrupt the microbiome. Like scented washes and douches, using scented tampons can impact pH. Sexual partners should always wash their hands and genitals with pH balancing cleansers before they get within five feet of your vagina.

Personal lubricants can make it easier to have an orgasm, and they can help our most sensitive skin (ten times as delicate as our facial skin) to avoid irritation and microtears during sex play. Just make smart choices about which lube to use, i.e., choose one that doesn't contain hazardous chemicals. Salted caramel-flavored lube might *sound* tasty, but waking up the next day with a burning infection isn't fun. Safe lubes should generally include those that are organic, scent-free, and water-soluble or silicone based. Oil-based lubes can potentially degrade latex condoms in just sixty seconds and have been associated with increased risk for bacterial vaginosis.[6]

Think twice about using condoms coated in spermicide. Granted, a condom does a good job at preventing pregnancy and reducing the spread of STIs. However, spermicide kills the beneficial bacteria in the vagina that keeps harmful strains and yeast in check. Some women might be allergic to spermicide and latex and not even know it. If you were allergic to, say, pineapple, your face might swell and your throat might close upon exposure. If you had a latex allergy, you wouldn't necessarily think of vaginal irritation and burning as an allergic reaction to a condom. "Women might be more sensitive to one brand or another," said Dr. Horton. "They should familiarize themselves with condom brands and types and, through trial and error, find out which ones are most comfortable for them and their vagina and keep their own stock on hand."

Sex toys—dildos, vibrators, and plugs—made from rubber or jelly can break down over time and store bacteria in their pores. Choose stainless steel or silicone sex toys instead, and wash them after every use with a fragrance-free, chemical-free pH-balanced personal care cleanser. You shouldn't clean sex toys with bar soap or scented washes.

A Smelly Vagina Is Not Necessarily Leaky

An entire industry was built around terrifying women into thinking their natural vaginal scent is offensive. The propaganda started in the early 1900s and hasn't let up since. In her book *Devices and Desires: A History of Contraceptives in America*, McGill history professor Andrea Tone reveals vintage ads from Lysol, the disinfectant company, that warned "wives" that their husbands were going to leave them because of their "objectionable odor" or "lack of intimate daintiness." By douching with Lysol disinfectant, wives could "destroy germs and odors," get "a clean, fresh, wholesome feeling," and regain their "dainty feminine allure" to win back their husbands' affections. The text in one ad reads, "Often a wife fails to realize that doubts due to one intimate neglect shut her out from happy married love." Sowing fear and doubt for a profit. From 1911 to 1952, the key ingredient in Lysol's feminine cleanser was the chemical cresol that caused severe burning, inflammation, and even death for some users.[7]

Your partner is not going to leave you because your vagina doesn't smell like Lysol (if they do, that's *not* a person you want to be with). Advertising that suggests they will do so preys on women's insecurities and is painfully effective. Men aren't conditioned to worry about that; a guy doesn't equate his own crotch smelling funky with a moral flaw or fear that it'll lead to divorce. He just takes a shower.

We need to rebrand women's concept of being clean and fresh down there. It's not soaping to the point of irritation and infection. It's not about smelling like lavender, fresh linen, or a summer's day. It's about smelling like *you*.

You might not smell the same day after day. Women's natural scent changes due to stress, and also hormonal and pH fluctuations during menstruation.[8] You might smell stronger after a workout or if you've been wearing clothing that doesn't breathe. That's totally normal.

"Every day, patients ask me what their vagina should smell like," said Dr. Horton. "What I tell them is, 'a healthy vagina smells like a vagina.'" Its scent is like no other, earthy, spicy, musky, sexy. A foul-smelling vagina—fishy, gassy, rotten—can be a sign of a bacterial imbalance, infection, or disease, or that a tampon was forgotten about and left inside. "Don't mask a foul smell with perfume or a drugstore douche," said Dr. Horton. "That'll only make it worse. Go to your doctor instead to discuss your options."

Fluids Aren't a Sign of Leaky Vagina Either

You might have heard that the vagina is like a self-cleaning oven. It's more like an acid wash with an always-open faucet. The glands just inside the vaginal entrance produce fluids during sexual arousal. When you're not aroused and just going about your daily life, slippery mucus rains down from the cervix into the vagina constantly. The word mucus might sound gross, but it's your vagina's best friend (and I'll talk more about its benefits later). It supports the microbiome, maintains an acidic pH, and lubricates the vaginal walls and vulva to prevent dryness and microtears that could get infected. As fluid and mucus rain down from the cervix and pour across the vaginal walls and vulva, they slough off dead human and microbiome cells, stuff you don't want in there anyway. You might not love seeing a half-a-teaspoon of discharge in the gusset of your panties at the end of the day. But it's completely healthy and normal—and better out than inside you!

It pains me that women think their fluid is offensive. Women often post on the Love Club, the Love Wellness community forum, about the color, amount, and consistency of it. A friend of mine is so embarrassed by her fluid, she hides her underwear in a separate laundry bag so her boyfriend will never know how much she produces per day. Discharge shame goes as far back as those Lysol ads from the early 20th century. But using products to "wash" the vagina interferes with the perfectly designed cleaning system we evolved to have. The irony is that using chemicals to wipe away fluid or mask smell may throw off your vaginal health, which could bring a strong odor and more copious and unhealthy discharge with it.

During pregnancy, it's common to have an increase in discharge. "It happens because of higher levels of progesterone, increased blood flow to the area, and increased cervical production of mucus," said urogynecologist Shweta Desai, MD, a Love Wellness medical advisor. The more mucus is produced, the more acid washing of pathogenic microbes takes place that might otherwise harm mother and baby.

Vagina-Adjacent Leaks: The Urinary Tract

The urinary tract is yet another body part that has its own microbiome. It's quite similar—but not identical—to the vagina's, and perhaps even more sensitive to leaks. The most common bacterial infection in humans occurs in the urinary tract. In women, urinary tract infections (UTIs) account for nearly 25% of *all* infections, 7 million doctor visits, 1,000,000 ER visits, and 100,000 hospitalizations per year.[9] I envy any woman who doesn't experience a UTI in her lifetime, but nearly half of us will.[10] For some of us, such infections happen with depressing frequency. I don't mention the D-word casually. Recurrent UTIs (one or more within six months) increase the risk for depression in sufferers.[11]

The basic biology of the urinary tract starts at the top with the kidneys, located on either side of your spine, just below the ribs. They are bean-shaped filters that clean your blood, remove waste, and turn it into urine. Urine drains from the kidneys through long tubes called ureters into the bladder, a muscular sac tucked into the pelvis between the uterus and the pelvic bone. When the bladder is full, we feel the urge to pee. After we voluntarily relax our bladder sphincter muscle, urine drains through a tube called the urethra, out through the urethral opening, the pee hole located between the clitoris and the vaginal opening, into the toilet or onto the forest floor, side of the road, or what have you.

UTI symptoms are unforgettable. According to the National Institutes of Diabetes and Digestive and Kidney Diseases[12] (and me), they include pain or burning when urinating, the urge to urinate often regardless of how much comes out, pressure in your lower abdomen, and off-smelling, milky, cloudy, or bloody urine. If you have a fever, too, it means the infection has reached the kidneys, which is cause for alarm and a trip to the emergency room. Older women with UTIs can experience fatigue, confusion, general shakiness, and weakness.

UTIs are caused by bad bacteria, often from the gut, getting into the urinary tract. The most prevalent culprit is *Escherichia coli*,[13] the bacteria in the news whenever there's a boxed lettuce recall. *E. coli* stealthily makes its way from the anus, across the vulva, into the urethra, and up into the bladder, without you having a clue until a day or two later when you start to pee fire.

"Women get eight times more UTIs than men due to the basic female anatomy," said Dr. Horton. "The urethral opening on a man is at the tip of the penis, which is nowhere near the anus. A woman's urethra and vagina are very close to the anus. The urethra itself on a woman is extremely short, just one-and-a-half inches. A male urethra is seven or eight inches. *E. coli* has a lot less travel distance in women to get into the bladder, adhere to the wall, and cause an infection."

A thirty-six-year-old friend of mine has recurrent UTIs; at least two every six months. "I get a UTI just looking at a condom," she said. "I am so careful. I wipe front to back religiously. I pee after sex, every time. I drink tons of water. And still, I live on the edge of anxiety about when I'm going to feel that first sign of pressure that means the pain is going to start soon. It's the worst feeling in the world. And then I have to go on antibiotics, which always winds up giving me diarrhea, which means more obsessive front-to-back wiping, and fear of contamination. It would be funny, if it weren't so tragic."

I feel for her and anyone who has chronic conditions. I have been there, and I know how awful the dread is, on top of the self-blame and the physical pain. "Drinking fluids to flush out the bladder and careful hygiene are important," said Dr. Horton. "But sometimes UTIs happen despite being conscientious. It's your body, but it's not your fault." Besides sex and vagina microbiome disruptors, other risk factors for UTIs are stress, inflammatory foods (curse you, gluten!), diabetes, pregnancy, and menopause.

The only treatment for a UTI is prescription antibiotics. You have to stop the infection in the bladder, because once it gets into the kidneys, you will need to be hospitalized and given antibiotics intravenously. Many women who have experience with UTIs will call their doctor and get a prescription over the phone. This can be dangerous because, without testing a urine sample for the specific type of infection, you might wind up taking an ineffective drug. Some bacteria are resistant to certain medications. If you take the wrong antibiotic, you could kill off beneficial bacteria without making a dent on the pathogenic one that caused the infection. Make sure you take the right medication by insisting on a urine test. And while you are on the correct antibiotics, consider also taking a probiotic supplement to help maintain a healthy microbiome.

In the next chapter, I'll go deeper on how these three parts communicate and connect via three specific pathways: the nervous system, the immune system, and the endocrine system.

LEAKY VAGINA

Here are some recommendations to help support vagina and urinary tract health:

TO-DO

- Learn the names of all your parts. If you know their names and can say them out loud, you can better describe problems to a doctor and get the care you deserve.

- You're taking a gut probiotic supplement that can support good bacteria everywhere, and another that is made for brain health and mood. Layer on another probiotic that's tailored to women's health—with multiple strains of *lactobacilli*—that can maintain normal acidity levels and promote a healthy microbiome in your vagina.

- Pack another bikini. Wearing damp clothing can increase the risk of yeast infections; your mother was right to tell you not to sit around in a wet bathing suit.

- Buy your own condoms. A guy might get the cheapest ones available or use one that's been in his wallet for six months. It might seem unfair that we have to deal with that, too, but being in control of everything that goes into your vagina can prevent infections that become much bigger burdens than buying condoms.

chapter 5

PATHWAYS

The gut, brain, and vagina have a partnership, where one keeps the others healthy, and vice versa (times three). These three parts, in three locations, in three systems, are in constant communication with one another and influence how each other functions.

Correspondingly, there are three pathways that keep them in touch: the nervous system, the immune system, and the endocrine system. By learning how the GBV axis hums along on these pathways and how to keep them clear of obstruction, you can optimize your health from top to bottom.

The Nervous System Pathway

From your own lived experience, you already know that the gut and brain are linked. You feel emotions in your gut, just as you feel them in your brain. In fact, sometimes your gut feelings might be even more accurate than your head feelings. Unlike your thinking, reasoning, rationalizing brain with its stored memories and psychological baggage, your gut reacts purely to what's happening in the moment. A good example: During my health mystery, my head was working overtime to rationalize my doctors' insistence that my issues were emotionally based. But deep down, my gut was telling me that something was wrong with me on a physiological level. My gut was eventually proven right.

While bonding with loved ones, you get a warm gooey sensation deep inside. Excited gut feelings might feel like butterflies in your belly. A sudden, upsetting incident might give you a sinking feeling in your stomach. The gut's emotional reactiveness is one of the reasons it's referred to as "the second brain."

The biological reason for why we "feel" things in the second brain is that the gut is packed with neurons (nerve cells). The entire central nervous system—the brain and the spinal cord—has 86 billion neurons. The enteric nervous system in your gastrointestinal system has 500 million neurons,[1] five times as many as in your spinal cord. In addition to the human neurons in the gut, the microbiome of trillions of cells has a vast nervous system of its own. If you want to get philosophical about it, each one of us contains a multitude of tiny brains that are reacting to their environment and circumstances every second of every day.

The brain in your head does the thinking, memorizing, theorizing, dreaming, learning, all the cognitive and creative stuff that makes life interesting. The brain's utilitarian jobs are controlling organ functions, making muscles move, and producing neurotransmitters—chemicals that hop across the synapses (gaps) between neurons, acting like mail carriers to deliver messages throughout the body.

The second brain, in your gut, controls digestion, hunger, and metabolism, and it receives and sends messages to brain number one. If your upstairs neurons send the message, "I'm hungry," to your downstairs neurons, your stomach steps up the production of gastric acid. When the downstairs brain sends the message, "I'm too full to eat another bite," to the brain upstairs, it tells you to put down the fork. If your first brain is scared, it wires down to the gut, and you get that heart-in-throat feeling. If your gut is stressed out, from a cortisol flood or a microbiome disruption, your brain will get antsy. Same thing if your gut is happy, balanced, and content. Your brain enjoys the quiet calm.

Previously, I mentioned bacterial cross-talk—the phenomenon where microbiomes in the gut and vagina, for example, text each other via chemical signaling. The brain doesn't have a microbiome, so that form of communication with the gut is off the table. No problem! The gut, brain, and microbiome chat directly via our biological equivalent of fiberoptic cable, namely the incredible vagus nerve.

You've Got Some Nerve!

The word *vagus* looks like vagina, but not because the vagus nerve (VN) is in the birth canal. (It isn't.) Vagus is Latin for "wanderer," and the VN lives up to that name. The longest nerve in the body not contained within the spinal column, the VN originates in the brain stem's medulla oblongata, divides into two branches that wrap around your throat, and ramble down from there. Every organ that you need to survive (and can think of, really!) is wired into the brain via the VN.

The wanderer nerve's main job is to relay messages back and forth between the brain and the body. Twenty percent of the VN's fibers are *efferent*, meaning the messages exit the brain and head down to your vital organs. If you are exercising, for example, the brain sends a message to the heart that says, "beat faster!" to increase blood flow to the muscles. When you eat a tuna sandwich, your brain tells the stomach to "send in the enzymes!" so you'll be able to break down the food into nutrient component parts.

Eighty percent of the VN's fibers are *afferent*, meaning the messages flow upstream from the organs to the brain. If your gut neurons and the brain trust of the microbiome detect border wall breaches, they report to the brain, "It's getting leaky in here! Send in the clean-up crew!" Because messages are both sent and received along the VN, your brain(s) can keep tabs on everything that's going on in your body, and other vital organs can let the brain know how they're doing and what they need.

If the VN's two-way fibers are strong, its lines of communication are open, and all outgoing and incoming messages are clear. However, the VN can be weakened, and then its messages between the brain and the body can get muddled. Miscommunication can destroy a relationship. Mixed signals with a boss can get you fired. When your brain and body communication system is jammed, one part doesn't know what the other is doing. As a result, your senses of hunger and satiety get scrambled, your immune response can go haywire, and your metabolism can slow to a crawl.

What weakens the VN? Let's focus on the usual suspects: inflammation[2] and stress. People with inflammatory bowel disease (IBD), IBS, and gut dysbiosis (microbiome imbalance) often have weak vagal tone as well. But when they stimulate their VN and improve its tone, the production of damaging inflammatory chemicals, cytokines, is inhibited[3] and microbiome balance can be restored.[4] So even if your VN is in bad shape because of chronic inflammation, strengthening it can also help de-puff your insides. It's a huge win-win.

I never get tired of saying, "It's all connected." When one part works, the others do, too. When the fiberoptic cable that connects the brain, gut, and microbiome is in good shape, it can help to seal leaks, tamp down internal swelling, and find body balance. But, if any part of this communications network is damaged, the whole system can go down.

Stress is another known VN weakener. When we experience emotional stress (feeling overwhelmed, burned out, or upset) and/or physical stress (from extreme exercise or disease), our adrenal glands release the stress hormones cortisol and adrenaline. Cortisol erodes the gut wall's protective mucus coating where your good bacteria live, weakening VN communication. At every point along the GBV axis, and as we've seen in the previous chapter, stress makes a mess.

Stopping stress before it starts is an excellent strategy for supporting wellness and maintaining microbiome balance. It can even help to prevent GBV axis leaks. But even Tibetan monks who meditate with singing bowls for ten hours a day can't always do that. Modern life is *full* of stressors, like nonstop video work calls, worrying about the person who is possibly ghosting you, and that bill coming due. We could tell ourselves, "It's going to be okay!" But it won't help if we're already panicking and the cortisol is flowing.

However, it is possible to cycle through the stress response faster and limit its ill effects by stimulating the VN. It's a huge bio-hack that we all need to learn to support our microbiome and our whole-body wellness plan.

Lightning-fast biology lesson: Our autonomic (involuntary) nervous system runs on two parallel tracks. One is the sympathetic nervous system (SNS), aka fight-or-flight response. The SNS kicks in whenever we perceive a threat—a car horn, a text that says you've reached your credit card limit—even if we're not in immediate life-or-death danger. In response, the adrenal glands release stress hormones, which immediately increase our heart rate, blood pressure, and respiration. The body redirects all our energy to our muscles so we can flee or fight, and nearly every other body function slows or stops. Bladder control stops working in fight-or-flight mode, which is why terrified people pee themselves. Pupils dilate. The vagina and uterus contract. As the brain is deprived of blood and oxygen in this state, we're not too smart when stressed and might do stupid things. Important life lesson: Do *not* send emails or call an ex when surfing a cortisol wave.

During my health mystery, I flowed from one cortisol flood to the next. My body rarely got the chance to calm down enough to shift out of fight-or-flight mode and into the autonomic nervous system's *second* track, the parasympathetic nervous system (PNS), aka "rest and digest." It kicks in whenever you feel relaxed and safe. Heart rate, blood pressure, and respiration slow down. Energy is directed into the digestive and urinary tracts. The vagina and uterus unclench. "Rest and digest" is also called "safe and social" because of the release of calming neurochemicals that put you in the mood for bonding and sex.

You can't be stressed and calm at the same time, just as you can't simultaneously run from a charging rhino and nap under a shady tree. Every minute of the day, we are either "on," in stress mode; or "off," in peace mode.

Here's a mnemonic device to help you remember the difference between the SNS and PNS parallel tracks: SNS starts with S for stress; PNS starts with P for peace. When your body is on the stress track, your GBV axis is at its worst. When your body is on the peace track, your GBV axis is at its best.

The VN, the nerve that runs through all of our GBV axis organs, just so happens to be the toggle switch between the SNS stress track and the PNS peace track. If you're already flooded with cortisol, stimulating the VN can exit the fight-or-flight mode faster. Since continued stress is a major cause of GBV axis leaks, shutting down stress and activating calm allows your body to love itself, reach homeostasis, and help you to heal without stress reactions.

Give Your Vagus Nerve Some Love

If I'd known I had the capacity to flip the calm switch to quiet my racing heart during my panic attacks, I would have been stimulating and toning my VN for hours a day. Nowadays, I'm mindful about it, practicing at least one of these techniques daily:

- COLD THERAPY. Splashing your face and neck with cold water can improve vagal tone.[5] The brave can try standing under an ice-cold shower for a minimum of thirty seconds daily to get VN boosting benefits.

- DEEP BREATHING. "Parasympathetic breathing" is instantly calming, even in extremely stressful situations. To follow this method: (1) inhale through the nose and into the belly for a count of four, (2) hold the breath for a count of seven, (3) exhale through the mouth for a count of eight. Repeat until you feel calmer.

- BUZZING. Activate the vocal cords to perk up the VN neck branches. OM chanting,[6] humming, gargling, chanting, or singing can tone the VN, increase calm, and lower the heart rate.[7]

- ACUPUNCTURE. If you haven't tried acupuncture yet, now is the time. Tiny needles inserted into head and neck acupoints stimulate[8] and tone[9] the VN.

- YOGA. British researchers had subjects practice different yoga poses to test if they had an impact on energy and self-esteem. Doing chest opening power poses for two minutes improved the subjects' energy and confidence—and improved vagal tone.[10]

- MASSAGE. Research from Taiwan found that reflexology massage of the feet increased vagal tone and decreased blood pressure in healthy subjects *and* those with coronary artery disease. You don't have to be a massage therapist to get benefits, just rub your own feet, stroke the sides of your neck, or ask your favorite person to do it for you.

- SOCIALIZING. Shifting into "safe and social" mode turns off stress and turns on positive emotions. A well-known study about the "upward spiral dynamic" of social engagement found that "increased positive emotions produced increases in vagal tone, an effect mediated by increased perceptions of social connections."[11] When you feel a sense of belonging, your VN function—and overall wellness—goes up.

- LAUGHTER. Laughter, especially with people you enjoy and care about, can increase positive emotions, happy hormones, and vocal cord buzzing, which are all contributing factors to a balanced microbiome and strong VN.

- HEALTHY DIET. Foods that are rich in omega-3 fatty acids (fish, healthy oils, greens, nuts, and seeds), zinc[12] (greens, nuts, seeds, and oysters), and probiotics[13] (yogurt and fermented foods) strengthen the VN and keep its lines of communication open.

- SEX. Speaking of . . .

The Third Brain

Oh, vagina, I haven't forgotten about you.

There are many women who would say that they "think with their vagina," and make decisions based on their sexual desires. We have all been there (and done that). I have not found any scientific research that proves the vagina can actually think. It definitely *feels*, though. The clitoris has 8,000 nerve endings (twice the number the penis has). The female reproductive tract is wired directly into the central nervous system via branches of the spinal cord. The three major vagina-brain nerves are (1) the clitoris's pudendal nerve, (2) the vagina's pelvic nerve, and (3) the cervix's and uterus's hypogastric nerve.

Another important nerve connects the genitalia to the brain *without* going through the spinal cord. It's our old, dear wanderer friend, the vagus nerve.

The VN is so long, it stretches low and deep enough into the abdomen to reach the uterus and the cervix. Vaginal penetrative sex with cervical stimulation with a penis or a toy strengthens the VN and supports the entire GBV axis. Even more exciting news: Cervical VN stimulation *alone* can make you have an orgasm.[14]

What better reinforcement of the vagina-brain axis do you need than that? Optimizing our health and having enjoyable sex can help make us feel good, in many wonderful ways.

The Immune System Pathway

The immune system is downright philosophical. It asks, *Who am I? What is the self? Who is not me? What is not the self? How do I know who I am?* Tough questions. Most of us would be hard pressed to answer them.

Our body's frontline defenders confront existential questions whenever a *not-self* substance gets into the body through a cut in the skin, crosses the gut or vaginal wall, or is inhaled into the lungs. As every breath we take brings in some *not-self* molecules, our immunity defenders are very busy. The microbiome is *not-self*. In a sealed gut, the microbiome stays within the gut walls (aka the doughnut hole) and doesn't cross over into the body (the doughnut). When microbes leak through the gut wall, their status changes from free riders to hostile invaders, and then they are met by the immune system response army.

The immune system is made up of organs, tissues, white blood cells, and proteins that all work together to fight our battles for us. Important immunity organs are the thymus, bone marrow, the spleen, and tonsils, which either produce or store (or both) immunity foot soldier white blood cells. The gut is an all-star immunity organ, blocking harmful stuff from getting into the body, trapping pathogens in its mucus layer, and secreting three to five grams of antibodies into the intestine every single day.[15]

The immunity army, in brief, is composed of white blood cells like leukocytes that circulate via the blood stream and lymphocytes that circulate via the lymphatic vessels; VIP lymphocytes, including T cells produced by the thymus and B cells produced in the bone marrow; and antibodies that are are Y-shaped blood proteins that target specific antigens (viruses, germs, and bacteria) and remember how to fight them in case they invade again. We develop immunity to a particular virus because our antibodies have a long memory. If we defeat an infection, we can develop resistance to it.

As soon as antigens get into the body, nearby cells (human and bacteria) send out a chemical alarm: "We're under attack!" White blood cells and antibodies heed the call and rush to the site of the issue. First, they determine if the substance is *self* or *not-self*. If it is *self*, our defenders stand down. If it's *not-self*, white blood cells attack and antibodies scroll through their memory banks to remember which weapons to use to kill the antigen that can cause an infection. If the immune response isn't savage enough, the virus or bad bacteria can get a foothold and cause an infection that needs extra help from specific antibiotics to conquer it.

The system works incredibly well, but it doesn't work perfectly. For example, our immunity defenders might launch an attack when we are exposed to a harmless food or chemical. Allergic reactions are basically unprovoked attacks that get out of hand. I mean, throat and face swelling from a peanut? Or dust? That's an overzealous inflammatory response.

Another imperfect immune response is when our defenders fail to recognize an attack from within. Defenders patrol the body for foreign invaders, not human cells that mutate and then multiply into a tumor. Even though the tumor can do us harm, the immunity cells still think it's *self* and therefore not a threat. That miscalculation can allow a malignancy to grow unheeded and spread into the lymphatic system and all over the body.

Almost the opposite of cancer, autoimmune disorders happen because, during a prolonged battle, in the fog of war, antibodies get confused about what is *self* and what's *not-self* and wind up attacking everything in sight, including healthy human cells. Autoimmune conditions are the result of friendly fire when the immune system attacks *auto*, the self. Many such illnesses have been associated with leaky gut. Which came first, the autoimmune issues or the gut leaks? The science is still pending. We do know that if you have one, you're likely to have gut leaks; and if you have gut leaks, the odds of having a friendly fire condition go up.

Got Lymph?

You might think that the lymphatic system of nodes and vessels is part of the circulatory system. Correct. In that system, the heart pumps blood through a network of arteries and veins. Right alongside it, lymphatic vessels carry lymph—a clear, plasma-like fluid—throughout the body in an independent, circulatory network. (You know lymph: When you go hiking for miles in new boots, the blister on your heel is filled with it.) Without a pump, lymphatic vessels rely on valves and muscle contractions to make sure the fluid keeps moving in the right direction. We can help lymph along with massage, bouncy exercise, and dry brushing.

The lymphatic system is a major part of the immune system as well. Your 500+ lymph nodes are scattered in singles or chains throughout the body, most prominently in your neck, above the collar bone, and in the armpits, chest, abdomen, and groin. These compelling little beans do the massive job of filtering toxins, germs, and viruses from circulating lymph. When nodes catch a ton of the bad stuff, they swell. You know how doctors feel your neck and armpits when you're sick? They are looking for swollen nodes, a symptom of an ear, sinus, or throat infection, and a sign that your natural defenses are not up to the task. Specific antibiotics will pick up where nodes left off.

Give Your Immune System Some Love

Certain lifestyle and dietary choices damage your immune system. Some things you can do are cut back on alcohol, smoking, refined sugar and flour, hydrogenated fats and oils, artificial sweeteners, food dyes, and preservatives. Also, move (for) your bowels. Gentle movement, though. Overexercise is counterproductive. The tipping point, according to a meta-review of the data, is two hours of intense exertion.[16] If you gasp for breath, you're going too hard. I don't recommend strenuous exercise while focusing on balancing the gut because it triggers gut-associated lymphoid tissue (GALT)-eroding cortisol floods. Low intensity walking and yoga reduce stress, tone the vagus nerve, and balance the gut.

I'm not saying you can't have fun! It's a balancing act, and no one is perfect. It's just about becoming more aware of how what goes into your body affects you. Vitamins, minerals, lean protein, healthy fats, and adequate hydration (eight to ten glasses of filtered water or herbal tea per day) support the production of white blood cells, antibodies, and lymphatic fluid. Help your inner army defend you against infection by ingesting these nutrient-dense foods:

- Brown and white rice, quinoa, and oatmeal
- Citrus fruits
- Dark fruits and berries
- Goat and sheep milk cheeses
- Green vegetables
- Herbs and spices including thyme, oregano, garlic, ginger, clove, basil, rosemary, onion, turmeric
- Legumes
- Organic eggs and chicken
- Organic flax oil, coconut oil, olive oil
- Organic grass-fed meats
- Wild fish

It's About Slime

You might even call it gross or disgusting, but we are nothing without mucosal tissue on our internal passages. "Mucus is an integral piece of the puzzle of our immune system," said Dr. Grosman. "I think of it as the bouncer. It has pores to let some things into the body [like water and nutrients], but it tells other things [like antigens] to go to the back of the line, and then never lets them in."

The entirety of the body's slime coating is called mucosal-associated lymphatic tissue (MALT). Seventy to eighty percent of our antibodies are produced and reside in the MALT. When the MALT is under attack from germs, mucus production increases to flush them out. You probably curse mucus when it flows like a broken faucet out of your nose when you have a cold, but that pile of tissues is actually evidence that your body is working hard to make you better.

The MALT has many subsections with punchy acronyms like the NALT (nasal-associated lymphoid tissue), SALT (skin-associated lymphoid tissue), and CALT (conjunctival-associated lymphoid tissue). Each subsection of mucus has its own characteristics and viscosity. For example, the mucus that keeps your eyeballs moist is thin and watery so you can blink. The mucus in your stomach is hardy and thick because it's bombarded with gastric acids. The small intestine's mucus is porous, so nutrients can be transported across it. In the lungs, mucus has the consistency of hair gel, just slippery enough to prevent bad bacteria from clumping and causing an infection[17] but not so thick that we can't breathe.

I'm mainly concerned with the MALT's two GBV-axis subsections, the GALT (gut-associated lymphoid tissue) and the VALT (vulvovaginal-associated lymphoid tissue).

The GALT

The GALT is your best friend. It has two tiers: a looser outer layer that is home to our trillions of microscopic friends and a tighter layer underneath that acts like a protective sealing wax for the gut wall, making sure everything moves safely and painlessly. If not for gut mucus, even the basic act of pooping could injure and inflame.[18]

What Does the GALT Do for You?

- **IT'S A SPONGE.** As nutrients are broken down in the stomach and small intestine, they are absorbed by the spongey mucus layer, transported across it, and ushered into the bloodstream.

- **IT LUBRICATES.** Mucus is the body's self-producing moisturizer, keeping your inner skin supple and smooth. If it were to dry out, it would crack, giving bad bacteria crevices to grow in. Additionally, you wouldn't be able to swallow or poop without it.

RETHINK YOUR "I'M ON VACATION!" EATING PLAN: A diet high in fat and simple sugars and low in fiber negatively impacts the GALT. Swedish researchers tested the effects on mice and found that exposure to a Western-style diet for just three days altered the subjects' microbiota composition, and their mucus layer got thinner and more porous.[19]

- **IT PROTECTS.** Mucus is a barrier that, in a sealed gut, prevents anything other than nutrient molecules and water from getting through the gut wall. Toxins and germs trapped by the GALT are then swept up by sticky mucus-coated feces and sent down the slippery slope of your colon, out the anus, and into the toilet.

- **IT'S HOME.** The GALT is your microbiome's sticky, cozy home. With a safe place to nestle, good bacteria can go about their business of living, reproducing, aiding your digestion, and boosting your immunity.

The GALT feeds the microbiome. Bacteria doesn't just eat prebiotic fiber. It also has a hankering for mucus and, as a result, produces postbiotics like butyrate from consuming it. Butyrate in the gut sends a chemical signal to mucus generators in the epithelial layer to step up production. To sum it up: Bacteria live in mucus, eat mucus, poop on mucus, and the poop makes more mucus. An equivalent would be if you ate your house, and in so doing, got a bigger, safer house.

If Your GALT Is Strong . . .

- You rarely get sick
- You can recover quickly from colds

- You can have loads of energy
- Your allergic reactions are often slight or nonexistent

- You can maintain adequate vitamin levels with a healthy diet

The GALT is vulnerable to degrading from poor diet, stress, inflammation, aging, and an imbalanced microbiome. "With a weak GALT, nutrients will pass through your gut like water, or what I call 'expensive urine,'" said Dr. Francis. To strengthen the GALT, she recommends supplementing with mucilaginous herbs, such as marshmallow, aloe, slippery elm, cat's claw, and licorice (pay attention to serving size; don't overdo it!).

If Your GALT Is Weak . . .

- You're likely prone to colds and flu
- You seem to take forever to get over an illness

- You always feel tired
- You likely suffer from allergies

- You probably have nutrient deficiencies
- You might have an autoimmune disorder

The VALT

If you thought the GALT was impressive, just wait until you hear about the VALT.

It must be said first that the vagina wall's immunity has not received the same attention in the research community as the gut's. When you read scientific papers on the subject, and I've read a lot, most of them start with some disclaimer like, "Our understanding of immune responses in the female reproductive tract has traditionally lagged behind our grasp of the situation at other mucosal sites . . ."[20] Mucus is yet another area of female health that gets shortchanged.

What makes the female reproductive tract (FRT) immunity so amazing is that it does everything the GALT does—like moisturize, protect, and house the microbiome—and so much more. The vagina's one-two punch of acid and mucus does a great job of natural defense against yeast infections.[21] The VALT's immunity T cells can help fight off chlamydia,[22] and its "natural killer cells" can lower the odds of contracting genital herpes[23] and human papilloma virus-related cervical cancer.[24] That said, we all are at risk of these STIs and our immunity is never perfect.

The VALT's immunity army has to be smart enough to make special exceptions to the *self* vs. *not-self* classification system. It knows that leaky vagina issues are *not-self* and attacks. But when it detects the presence of certain *not-self* substances, like semen, it stands down. If the VALT's immunity foot soldiers always rushed to kill sperm immediately upon detection—and they could if they wanted to—the human race would cease to exist. Not only does sperm get a hall pass to travel freely in the vagina, through the cervical gateway, into the uterus, and up the fallopian tubes where it might meet an egg and fertilize it, the VALT actually helps sperm on its way. During ovulation, cervical mucus alters itself, thinning to an egg-white consistency that allows sperm to glide along.[25] The mucus change and the FRT immune cells lowering their guard creates a "window of opportunity" for conception. However, it can simultaneously create a "window of vulnerability" for contracting STIs.[26] Forewarned is forearmed.

A fertilized egg drops into the uterus, implants itself on the blood-lined wall, and its cells continue to divide rapidly until they grow into an embryo. That embryo is derived from a *self* cell (the egg), but the embryo is *not-self*. The VALT's immunity cells recognize that the embryo, and later, the fetus, is a foreign invader, but they let it hang out anyway for nine whole months. Meanwhile, the cervix mucus production ramps up during pregnancy and forms a plug that blocks any pathogens from getting near the fetus. Its concentration of killer antibodies and cytokines increases, too.[27] The cervix doesn't get the credit it deserves as an immunity organ.

As amazing as it is, the VALT is vulnerable to breakdown. I've included a bunch of tips in the following section to keep your VALT, well, a *vault*.

Give Your VALT Some Love

Drink plenty of water and eat foods that improve mucus quality, like greens, proteins, and healthy fats[28] that have been found to balance hormones. To step up VALT production, improve mucus quality, and (if it's important to you) support reproductive health, eat more of these foods:

- Omega-3 fatty acid foods like fish, nuts, seeds, and greens

- Plant proteins like tofu, beans, lentils, edamame, whole grains

- Zinc- and iron-rich vegetables like spinach, broccoli, bok choy, and leafy greens

- Vitamin B–rich whole grains, poultry, eggs, legumes, bananas, citrus fruits

THE ENDOCRINE SYSTEM PATHWAY

I visualize the complexity of the endocrine system of organs, glands (hormone factories), and hormones (chemical messengers) as an Amazon fulfillment center. Have you seen videos from inside one of those warehouses? Robots, drones, machinery, and humans are all moving rapidly in every direction. Yet, somehow, they don't crash into each other and manage to get the right goods in the right amounts into the right box with the right shipping label. Then the packages are shipped to the right destination and placed in the hands of the right recipient.

Your endocrine system manages to do all that for you. It produces many different hormones in glands and organs and sends them out to be delivered to the right receptors via the bloodstream, along with a set of instructions. It's organized chaos, but when the system works, our fifty-plus hormones are dispatched all over the body so each part functions exactly as it should. Our bones and muscles develop and grow. We get hungry and feel full. Food is converted to energy. Blood sugar stays under control. We respond to danger, get sleepy and wake up, feel desire, get aroused, love each other, get our periods, grow placentas, and go into labor. Hormones have a hand in *everything*. And each player on the GBV axis is a crucial endocrine organ.

The Brain's Hormone Factories

The pineal secretes melatonin, the sleep hormone that makes you feel tired. The hypothalamus is the time-keeper of our circadian rhythms. The pituitary "master gland" is only pea-sized but makes hormones that control other glands—and it helps to regulate pain!

The bow tie–shaped thyroid, appropriately located in the front of the neck, regulates bone growth when we're young and our metabolism (breaking down nutrients to turn into energy) throughout our lives. Its subglands, the parathyroids, help to regulate blood calcium levels.

The triangular adrenals aren't located anywhere near the brain—they sit on top of the kidneys—but they work with brain glands as an integral part of the hypothalamic–pituitary–adrenal (HPA) axis that helps to control our stress response, sex drive, cardiovascular system, immunity, and central nervous system.

The Vagina's Hormone Factory

The ovaries do double duty. As glands, they produce estrogen and progesterone—hormones that trigger puberty and regulate menstruation, pregnancy, and fountain-of-youth stuff like skin elasticity. As organs, at the time of our birth, they house a million follicles, each with an immature egg inside it. By puberty, that number drops to 300,000, and only about 300 of them will be released into the wild during a woman's menstruating decades. I love the trippy (but science-y!) truth that when we are fetuses in our mother's womb, we already contain in our teeny ovaries the egg that might one day become our daughter. So your mother wasn't only carrying her daughter, but her grandchild as well. How cool is that?

The Gut's Hormone Factories

The pancreas, part of our digestive system, stays very busy as an organ, producing bile to break down lipids. As a gland, it makes insulin, the hormone that regulates blood sugar.

The largest hormone-producing organ in the body is the gut itself.[29] Its tremendous number of enteroendocrine cells are spread throughout the GALT where they make and release dozens of hormones, such as ghrelin, sometimes called "the hunger hormone," that tells our brain it's time to eat, and gastrin that tells our stomach to release gastric acid in anticipation of eating. A key gut-brain axis hormone, leptin, often refered to as "the satiety hormone," sends messages from the gut to the brain to help signal to you that you've had enough.

Serotonin is often thought of as a brain hormone because it's closely related to the regulation of anxiety and depression, when in truth, the brain makes only 10% of our precious supply of serotonin. The other 90% is produced in the gut.[30] An abundance of research (see every previous chapter) links poor gut health with depression and anxiety and improvement of gut health with relief from those conditions. A happy gut makes more happy hormones. An unhappy gut makes us unhappy campers.

Beyond the gut's enteroendocrine cells, the microbiome's trillions of cells play a huge part in sending, delivering, and activating hormones. Even though the microbiome is *not-self* and does not share our DNA, our bacteria free-riders regulate the movement and timing of hormones throughout our bodies. They're like the supervisors in the Amazon warehouse of our endocrine system, each microbiota holding its own microscopic clipboard.

It is not an exaggeration to say that the microbiome is fully in charge of our endocrine system, and therefore it can influence everything we do. We are in many ways completely at the mercy of our bacteria.

The microbiome, which is not a part of us, is perhaps best referred to as our most important endocrine organ.

Bacteria: Our Hormone Whisperers

One paper I read about human-bacteria "interkingdom" communication said that it's only possible because we share a common language: hormones.[31] Hormones are like a translation app that allows us to understand bacteria and bacteria to understand us. Where we stand now, bacteria might be more fluent at speaking "hormone" than we are. They issue commands, like "more of that," "less of this," "step that up," and "slow that down," controlling the hormonal give and take that affects the functioning of our first, second, and third brains, and every organ in between. In a very real way, the microbiome controls its host's mood, cognition, and behavior.

The interkingdom communication between the microbiome and us is complex and is still somewhat mysterious, but scientists are working hard to figure it out.

Irish neuroscientists fed mice either *Bifidobacterium*—a probiotic—or the antidepressant Lexapro. Then, to test their stress levels, they put the mice into a water tank with smooth sides. (The mice were not allowed to drown, BTW; they were rescued before it got that far.) The probiotic was just as effective as Lexapro in keeping the mice's stress response under control.[32] Big picture, bacteria is involved in the regulation of cortisol. I'm not going to tell anyone not to take prescribed medication, but the science does show that probiotics help to tamp down anxiety, at least in mice.

In a follow-up experiment, researchers gave mice either *lactobacillus* or plain broth before putting them in a maze, and then checked their gamma-aminobutyric acid (GABA) levels. GABA, a neurotransmitter, regulates hormone secretion and helps calm you down when you're upset. The probiotic-treated mice had higher GABA levels, entered the maze in a four-paws-on-the-ground "ready" stance, stayed in the maze longer, and tried harder to solve it compared to the control group.[33]

Using this study as a metaphor for life, we are all standing at the entrance of a maze, and our success is determined to a large extent by our willingness, intention, and determination to get on all fours and find that cheese. Probiotics can put us in the right frame of mind to go for it.

I've got a human study, too, by neurobiologists at Oxford University. Their participants' cortisol levels were checked and then they were given prebiotics that feed *Lactobacillus* and *Bifidobacteria* or a placebo. Next, the subjects watched words pop up on a screen with obvious positive or negative connotations while their eye movements were tracked. Afterwards, their cortisol levels were checked again. The prebiotic group had lowered cortisol levels post-experiment, compared to the control group, and they focused more on positive language.[34]

The influence of bacteria is often quite direct. *Lactobacillus reuteri* in the gut regulates insulin. If levels of *L. reuteri* are insufficient due to a gut imbalance, blood sugar can become harder to control. *Lactobacillus rhamnosus*, a gut and vagina probiotic, produces an acid that can speed up metabolism (an endocrine function) and reduces body fat, regardless of what you eat.[35] With bacteria, it's always about striking the right balance. But keep in mind that sudden changes in mood, energy, and weight—without any obvious cause—don't *necessarily* mean that it is solely caused by emotional strife. They could very well be hormonal issues that can be exacerbated by a microbiome imbalance. Eating a lot of plant-based fiber to feed *L. rhamnosus* might be the weight control bio-hack you've been looking for.

The Perils of Hormonal Imbalance

Bacteria produce, metabolize, and regulate hormones that make us feel happy, healthy, and calm. They can produce gold nuggets like butyrate, acetate, and propionate that support key hormones that help with digestion and speed up metabolism. When the gut microbiome is healthy and balanced, your hormones are likely to be in balance, too. If everything is working as it should, you can feel great, sleep well, have a robust sex drive, and easily maintain your weight. I call that whole-body harmony.

If a microbiome imbalance throws hormones out of whack, the result is a whole-body breakdown, and then you're up *Schitt's Creek* without Dan Levy to paddle for you. Basically, if bacteria are unable to communicate to endocrine glands and organs, important messages can get dropped. One lost message in a system this complex can cause a chain reaction that could lead to countless miscommunications, and the organized chaos of a functional endocrine system can fall into dysfunctional just-plain chaos, affecting mood, sleep, metabolism, weight, libido, and hunger.[36] In the gut, hormonal balance is important to skin health, digestive health, and cognitive health. An imbalanced microbiome alters the amount of estrogen circulating in the body, which might contribute to various issues related to metabolic, cognitive, and heart health.

What causes hormonal imbalances? Many of the same factors that cause and exacerbate a microbiome imbalance. Continued stress, for example, can fatigue the adrenals and lower progesterone levels, which can impact brain health, the ability to sleep, mood, and reproductive health. Plus, it can sap the production and release of feel-good hormones like dopamine, serotonin, and adrenaline.

If we are not getting enough sleep, our hormone factories can't run at full capacity. That deficit limits melatonin secretion, so we don't feel sleepy when we should and wind up not getting enough sleep. If you can't sleep, you can't get into the factory. And if you can't get into the factory, you can't sleep. It's an impossible balance beam!

Also on that hormonal balance beam are dietary and environmental toxins. Guess what they can do? Exactly, they can knock you off. Endocrine disruptor toxins can be found in some pesticides, plastics, petroleum, nonorganic foods, body care, beauty products, and cleaning products. They're hard to avoid. Hormones are metabolized in the gut and liver, the same places where toxins are filtered and eliminated. The gut and liver can only do so much at a time, so if they are occupied clearing toxins, some hormones won't be adequately processed. I understand that some side effects of an overtaxed liver can include acne, cysts, headaches, mood disorders, and inflammation.

Rebalancing Act

Our complex messenger system can be easily broken, but it can also be supported so that it—and you—can thrive. Start where all good health begins: in the gut.

In a randomized study of healthy adults, half of the participants took a probiotic supplement for four weeks and half took a placebo for the same length of time. Before and after the study period, the participants were assessed on their susceptibility to "saddening cues" (say, a commercial with a Sarah McLachlan song and images of rescue dogs in cages) and rated on a depression sensitivity scale. Compared to the

GBV AXIS HORMONAL IMBALANCE SIGNS

Here's a chart based on my understanding of how it all works:

GUT	BRAIN	VAGINA
Weight gain	Anxiety	Premenstrual syndrome (PMS)
Constipation	Depression	Irregular cycles
Poor nutrient absorption	Fatigue/Insomnia	Fibroids and ovarian cysts
Blood sugar problems	Memory issues	Infertility
Chronic inflammation	Headaches	Menopause symptoms

control group, the probiotic group showed significantly reduced sensitivity to sadness, fewer aggressive thoughts, and less anxious rumination.[37] This is a huge deal! Probiotics can help to make you more balanced, and even help your mood in just a few weeks. Keep an eye out for a probiotic supplement with butyrate-producing *Faecalibacterium* and *Coprococcus* bacteria that have been consistently associated with higher quality-of-life indicators.[38]

Stress Is Coming for Your Vagina, Too

The vagina is just as susceptible to the ravages of cortisol as the gut and the brain. The very last thing you need when you're under pressure or threat is a raging vaginal infection. Unfortunately, in those circumstances the probability of that happening goes way up. Cortisol can disrupt vaginal pH, which is associated with dysbiosis and inflammation.[39] Stress might not start in the female reproductive or urinary tract, but it often winds up there.

Cortisol has a seesaw effect on estrogen. When cortisol goes up, estrogen goes down. Low estrogen can disrupt your menstrual cycle (which is why your period might be late when you're going through a rough time) and reduce vaginal/cervical lubrication. With a dust bowl between your legs, you probably won't be in the mood for sex. Decreased estrogen has been associated with low libido (not wanting it) and decreased arousal (poor blood flow to the genitals).

Your vulva holds the secret to ridding you of cortisol and getting back your hormonal balance. It's a simple matter of pressing (or stroking, etc.) your love button, the clitoris, and having an orgasm. This isn't theoretical or anecdotal. It's hormonal. Oxytocin, a stress-modulating hormone, is released by the pituitary gland during orgasms (and nipple play), sending cortisol levels plummeting. Even just thinking about sex—whether you have an orgasm or not—increases serotonin and dopamine.[40] Those feel-good hormones modulate cortisol, too, and can make you less stressed and happier.

The vagina might not be an endocrine organ, but it is a pathway through which we can access brain and gut hormones that change our outlook on life.

So far, I've explained GBV axis leaks, and how these three organs and the microbiome communicate via the nervous, immune, and endocrine systems. Now you have the "why exactly" to know what might be causing gut, brain, and vagina problems. The next part of this book is devoted to supporting GBV axis organs and streamlining the comms systems between them in order to get to optimal functioning.

Getting back to normal is possible with love and self-care—and science! By tending to your microbiome, you are loving yourself well.

PATHWAYS

The GBV axis organs work better individually and collectively when they can talk to each other and help each other out. To keep those lines of communication open, I recommend the following:

- Every day, practice a few techniques to tone the vagus nerve to switch out of damaging stress mode and get on the peace track. When your body is calm and relaxed, your gut, brain, vagina, and microbiomes are their happiest.

- Support your immune system now by cutting back on lifestyle choices—smoking, drinking, eating junk—that damage it.

- Keep your GALT strong and sticky by giving your microbiome the food it craves: plant fiber. The more prebiotics you eat, the more postbiotics your microbiome is likely to produce. And nothing ramps up mucus production quite like postbiotics.

- Keep your VALT strong and sticky. Minimize stress, eat plants, and maintain an acidic pH in the vagina by using chemical-free and unscented products.

- Taking gut, mood, and vagina probiotic supplements and prebiotic fiber can help to support your endocrine system and support your sleep, weight management, metabolism, desire, and mood. Bacteria regulate our hormones, and by taking care of the microbiome, they will take care of you.

LOVE YOURSELF WELL

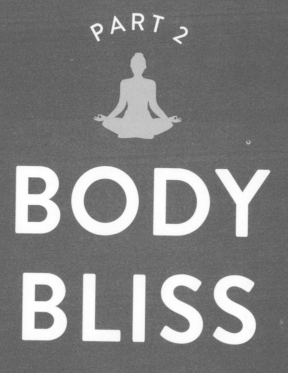

PART 2

BODY BLISS

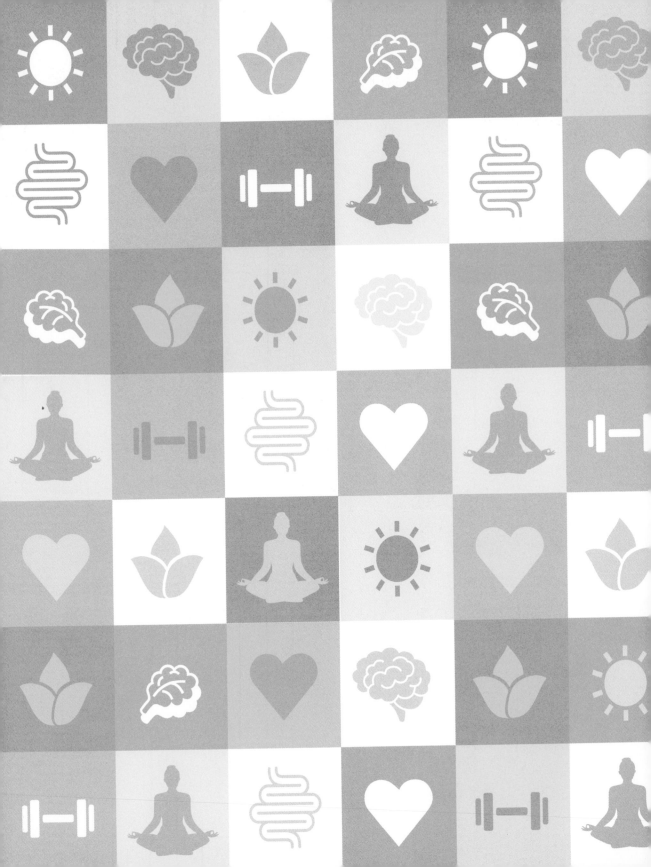

chapter 6

HAPPY GUT

I s your gut happy or cranky? You probably have powerful gut feelings on the subject, based on what's going on in your digestive tract right now.

But just to be sure, answer true or false to these statements:

1. In the last twenty-four hours, I have had a bowel movement that was so impressive, I almost took a picture of it. T or F

2. I could set my watch by how regular I am. T or F

3. Diarrhea is rare, and easily explained when it does happen. T or F

4. I get bloated only for a day or two before I get my period. But even then, it's not like I have to wear joggers to work. T or F

5. After I eat, I feel completely energized. T or F

6. My skin hasn't been this clear in years. T or F

7. I have to deal with the stress of modern life, but I wouldn't say that anxiety and depression are major concerns for me. T or F

8. I never get heartburn or indigestion. T or F

9. Constipation? Not a factor. T or F

10. Gas happens to us all, but mine isn't painful, too smelly, or embarrassing. T or F

11. I can eat pretty much anything without worrying about a bad reaction (gas, bloating, nausea, pain). T or F

12. After a meal, I feel satisfied and ready for action. T or F

If you answered "True" to eight or more statements, congratulations! I bet you have a happy gut that's probably leak-free and has a balanced microbiome. Your gut wall is probably doing its two main jobs: absorbing nutrients and blocking toxins from passing through. You can just skip ahead to the next chapter. (The rest of us, looking on jealously, will see you there.)

If you answered "False" to eight or more statements, you're telling me your gut is cranky and, based on what I've learned over the years, could be leaky. Digestive issues (occasional pain, bloating, constipation), food allergies and intolerances, skin conditions, and mood changes are the dead giveaways.

Most guts are likely to fall somewhere between happy and cranky, with seven or fewer "True" answers. In-the-middle guts deal with occasional bloating, gas, constipations, food that seems to just sit in your stomach, and feeling so tired after a meal that you want to lie down.

If you went to a gastroenterologist to see if you have leaky gut, you might be disappointed. Five years before my health mystery, in my late twenties, I had severe acid reflux. Ever the good patient, I went to a GI specialist to find out what was going on. He recommended an endoscopy. For this procedure, they inserted a flexible tube with a camera and a light into my mouth, snaked it down the throat, through the esophagus, into the stomach, and stopped at the duodenum, the entrance of the small intestine. Thankfully I was unconscious the whole time and didn't feel a thing.

When I woke up in the recovery room, the doctor said, "Everything looks fine."

"So why do I have such terrible acid reflux?"

"I don't know. It's probably due to eating acidic foods," he said. "Cut back on coffee and chocolate. Just take Tums when you have symptoms."

There was no discussion about the integrity of my gut wall, my microbiome, or whether the medications I was taking at the time (antibiotics and NSAIDs) may be contributing to my condition. The doctor could only go by what he saw. The endoscopy camera provided clear, enlarged images of my upper digestive tract, but it wasn't a microscope. The bacteria in the esophagus and stomach are invisible to the naked eye, and he never peeked in my colon, where most of the microbiome lives. Even if it had been visible, a sample would have had to have been tested to detect an imbalance. Apart from looking for obvious signs of gastroesophageal reflux disease (GERD), like an ulcer, the endoscopy was kind of pointless. I didn't know at the time (and I wonder if my doctor did) that what I was experiencing may be related to gut dysbiosis. Medications to treat GERD, like antacids (Tums) and proton pump inhibitors (Prilosec), have been associated with microbiome imbalances.[1]

In hindsight, I was likely dealing with a bacterial issue, but it was never brought up. I don't blame the doctor for not making the connection or mentioning the possibility. After all, who was talking about the microbiome in 2010?

Even now, Dr. Grosman tells me that gastrointestinal doctors are hesitant to recommend probiotics to their patients. The research is still new, and the microbiome is so complex. We know that some bacterial strains are beneficial, and some are pathogenic, that diversity is key, and that chronic antibiotics are like napalm in the gut. I was raised to believe that antibiotics were life-saving miracle drugs, and they absolutely are. But based on my own experience and what I understand, overuse can potentially devastate the gut, brain, and vagina.

Years later, when I learned about my dangerously low vitamin B and D levels, I naturally thought, "I really need to improve my diet." At the time, I relied a bit too heavily on premade foods and take-out. I didn't have a degree in nutrition, but I'd been to culinary school with a farm-to-table emphasis and was aware of the health benefits of fresh, organic food. I knew ideally I'd be eating that instead of processed and mass-produced stuff (even though usually that's a *lot* easier). Spurred to action, I shopped at the farmers' market and shifted toward eating local, seasonal produce and organic proteins I cooked myself. My diet was cleaner than it had been in years. I was eating forests of broccoli, getting vitamin B shots and taking vitamin D3 supplements . . . and it still wasn't enough to resolve all my health concerns. I was better, but not optimal; far from it. I was doing everything right, but I still felt lousy.

Here's the thing with a cranky gut: If you have leaks, it doesn't matter how clean you eat. If your mucus layer is degraded and the microbiome is imbalanced, nutrient absorption is compromised. A mountain of kale wasn't likely to fix me. To benefit from all that organic goodness I was eating, I had to make my way toward a healthy balanced gut *first*. Otherwise, I might as well dump my organic berries straight into the trash.

I would never tell anyone not to live their lives to the fullest. If bread makes you happy and you don't have a gluten sensitivity and leaky gut symptoms, go forth to the bakery. But if you *do* have a cranky, leaky gut, it's probably not going to magically turn happy until you are back to normal balance.

Happy Gut Goal #1: Balance

To help support a blissful state of gut homeostasis and harmony along the GBV axis, consider this equation:

PREBIOTICS + PROBIOTICS = POSTBIOTICS

I call it the "happy gut trifecta." In combination, I believe these three items are a really great way to support gut health, nutrient absorption, and a strong mucus layer, and to maintain tight junctions between the gut wall's epithelial cells. Let's go over them one by one.

PREBIOTICS

Prebiotics are soluble and insoluble fiber, aka indigestible carbohydrates, from plants.

Soluble fiber dissolves in water. In the digestive track, it turns into mush that soaks up water, which can bulk up poop and support its passage.

Insoluble fiber does not dissolve in water. It's called "roughage" because it exits the digestive track roughly the same way it entered. (I might have made up the etymology . . . but it works!)

You need both kinds of fiber for healthy elimination, and your gut bacteria feeds on both. But when good bacteria feast on soluble fiber, a process called "gut fermentation" kicks into high gear. After eating fiber, bacteria metabolize it into energy, and what's left over turns into metabolites, aka fermentation end products, aka postbiotics. Our human digestive process is very similar to that of our bacteria friends. We eat carbohydrates, convert them into energy, and whatever is left becomes another kind of (rear) end product.

Human fecal matter is comparable to bacterial postbiotics. The quality of our poop is determined by the food we eat. For example, if you eat a lot of roughage, your stool will achieve enviable quadruple S (smooth, soft, solid, and shapely) status. Remember how I mentioned earlier there's a whole industry devoted to selling admirable poop? If you hit quadruple S status, you're golden; you can make money with that poop. And here's a tip: Our microbiome makes high-quality end products after eating specific types of prebiotics, like inulin from vegetables and pectin from fruits. So if you're ready to get into that market, start with fruits and veggies.

Experts recommend consuming three to five grams of prebiotics per day to adequately feed your good bacteria. To hit that number, you can supplement with fiber gummies, powder, or pills. Most supplements' base ingredient is psyllium husk, and there's science to back up the fact that this supports a balance of the microbiome.[2] Another option is to grind flax seeds and sprinkle them liberally on everything as a delicious, potent prebiotic source.[3]

Or just eat more plants (you'll see a lot of these as ingredients in the recipes later in the book):

- APPLES. Full of the soluble fiber pectin, apples decrease gut inflammation and bad bacteria populations and yield a gold mine of short-chain fatty acids (SCFA) like butyrate.[4]

- ASPARAGUS. These green shoots support the GBV axis probiotic superstars *Bifidobacteria* and *Lactobacillus*.[5]

- BANANAS. Go for greenish-yellow unripe bananas for less sugar and more prebiotic fiber.[6]

- COCOA. Add cocoa powder to foods and beverages for delicious results, increased good gut bacteria, and decreased pathogenic bacteria.[7]

- DANDELION GREENS. A great source of antioxidants, they reduce blood sugar and inflammation, and regulate the immune system.[8]

- GARLIC. These smelly cloves make everything taste good, ward off vampires, boost the *Bifidobacteria*, and stunt the growth of pathogenic bacteria in the gut.[9]

- JERUSALEM ARTICHOKE. The fiber in sunchokes lowers cholesterol, aids the absorption of minerals in the colon, and supports overall digestive function.[10]

- LEEKS. Great in soups, grilled, or used as an onion substitute, this root vegetable is full of prebiotic fiber and vitamin K.

- OATS. Whole oats bring prebiotic fiber and support heart health.[11]

- ONIONS. The ultimate base ingredient, onions are natural antibiotics and antioxidants that help good gut bacteria flourish.[12]

PROBIOTICS

As you know (and if you don't, you really haven't been paying attention), probiotics are beneficial bacteria. They help to usher nutrients across the gut wall. As they're acidic, they can help support your immune system to control overgrowth of bad bacteria, yeast, and fungi that are not supposed to be there and could interfere with normal nutrient absorption. They can help to fortify the mucus layer, preventing toxins and germs from sticking to the gut wall or leaking through it. They can support the production of neurotransmitters that send signals to the brain and tell the gut wall muscles to contract and the enteroendocrine cells to make happy hormone serotonin.

Colloquially, when people say "probiotics," they are referring to supplements, capsules full of live strains of microorganisms like *Lactobacillus* and *Bifidobacterium*. Taking daily supplements replenishes the populations already living inside you that are otherwise struck down by stress, over-the-counter (OTC) medications, junk food, caffeine, and happy hour. Besides supplements, probiotics are found in food as well. Try to have one or two servings per day of the following:

- KEFIR. This milk drink, like yogurt, has added active cultures. As a probiotic food source, it might be better than yogurt because of its bacterial diversity.[13] Taste-wise, it's sour, like buttermilk, and not for everyone. If you can get used to it, kefir aids digestion and boosts immunity. (More about yogurt later.)

- KIMCHI. It's like sauerkraut . . . but spicy. The Korean cabbage dish contains a namesake probiotic called *Lactobacillus kimchii*. One study described kimchi as procolorectal health, probrain health, proskin health, and immunity supportive. There is nothing this side dish—or delicious ingredient in a meal—can't do.[14]

- MISO. Miso is made by fermenting soybeans with koji, a fungus. Eat it for the salty umami flavor, and get an abundant dose of vitamins and minerals with your probiotics.

- SAUERKRAUT. Fermented cabbage is rich in vitamins (B, C, K), minerals (iron, manganese), and probiotics.

- TEMPEH. It's like tofu . . . but fermented. This soy-based brick has loads of vitamin B12, which is usually only found in eggs, meat, and fish, making tempeh a great choice for vegetarians.[15]

- YOGURT. The difference between milk and yogurt is the additional lactic acid and *Bifidobacteria*, both probiotics. Check yogurt labels for the words "active cultures" or you'll wind up eating dead bacteria that does you no good.

POSTBIOTICS

And now we come to the end (products). Postbiotics are probiotic metabolites, bioactive compounds that come from gut fermentation. They include good stuff like bacteriocins (the body's very own antibiotics), enzymes (compounds that break down food), and postbiotic all-stars, SCFAs such as butyrate, acetate, and propionate.[16]

Why do I refer to SCFAs as gold nuggets? Because they help us live our best life. Here is some of what they can do for us:

- SUPPORT IMMUNITY. The SCFA butyrate can stimulate the production of immunity T cells that target pathogens and support a healthy immune system response.[17] They can also improve our ability to make antibodies to ward off antigens (germs and toxins).[18]

- SUPPORT MOOD. Butyrate has been associated with tightening the screws of loosened tight junctions in both the gut and the brain,[19] supporting mental clarity, brain health, and mood,[20] and supporting brain cell formation. I, for one, can always use some fresh brain cells, and having a well-fed microbiome appears to be one way to get them.

- MAINTAIN GI HEALTH. **Butyrate supplements that help to support your GI system can play a huge role in supporting overall health.**[21]

- MAINTAIN HEALTHY WEIGHT. **SCFA have been associated with suppressing hunger signals between the gut to the brain via our friend the vagus nerve.**[22]

- SUPPORT HEALTHY BLOOD SUGAR. **If you have a glucose sensitivity, eating more fiber might help support blood health and weight management.**[23]

Once the gut is healthy, by using the formula of prebiotics + probiotics = postbiotics for several weeks, you'll hopefully be absorbing nutrients in food like normal, have a healthy immune system, and be on your way to supporting your general health and well-being.

Happy Gut Goal #2: Support

If your gut is a castle, toxins are like enemies at the gates. If their numbers are overwhelming, eventually invaders are going to get in.

Limiting exposure is easier said than done, as environmental toxins are literally everywhere. Parabens are in our cosmetic products. Mold is in the walls. Heavy metals are in the water supply, lead paint, and treated wood. Phthalates are in plastic. Pesticides are sprayed on fruits, vegetables, and grain crops, and they aren't only on the plants, but in the soil the plants grow in. Commercially raised cows, pigs, chicken, and fish are fed pesticide-treated grains, antibiotics, and steroids. Whatever they eat, you eat. You might not take antibiotics and steroids, but if you eat commercially raised livestock, you ingest them just the same, and they damage your GALT and microbiome.

Steering toward organic foods, household products, and cosmetics products is a proactive strategy to support gut happiness, as those items won't erode your mucus or annihilate your friendly bacteria. By not making their job harder, they will thrive and show their gratitude to you by pumping out gold nuggets that make you feel great.

GO ORGANIC

The price difference between organic and nonorganic foods can be kind of shocking, I grant you. A pound of nonorganic carrots at my local supermarket is $1.59; the same size bag of organic carrots costs $2.29. If price is a factor (and when isn't it?), I've got some workarounds for you that will save you some money:

- Buy frozen organic fruits and veggies instead of fresh.

- Shop at a farmers' markets. Buying direct from growers shaves off the middle-man markup.

- Don't buy in bulk. Without preservatives, food goes bad quicker. Shop for just a day or two at a time.

- Buy dried legumes instead of canned. They're cheaper and safer. The lining in cans is coated with a resin containing bisphenol A (BPA), a synthetic estrogen that causes a hormonal imbalance.

- Join a food co-op. Food co-ops are worker- or customer-owned businesses that aim to sell the highest quality groceries, often from local growers, to members at bulk prices.[*]

While shopping at supermarkets, read the labels before buying anything. To get an official "organic" seal from the United States Department of Agriculture (USDA), I understand the product has to be certified to be 95% free of prohibited substances like harmful chemical pesticides and fertilizers. It's not perfect, but let's not let perfect be the enemy of the good. If a product is labeled "100% organic," it is probably a single ingredient item—a potato, a carrot—made without any trace of the government's list of prohibited substances. The USDA label "made with organic ingredients" means the product has cleared the 70% bar for organic ingredients.

Organic meat, poultry, eggs, and dairy products are raised/produced without growth hormones or antibiotics, and the animals that produce

---

[*]   Go to localharvest.org to find a food co-op near you.

them are fed only organic grain or grass, so I look for the label "hormone and antibiotic free." "Free range" sounds good, like the animals were romping in meadows among the wildflowers, but it doesn't mean anything. "Pasture raised" is dubious because it means that the animal had access to a pasture at some point in its life, maybe for just one day. For that matter, "natural" does not mean "organic." The language is intentionally confusing to get you to buy it. Don't take the bait!

Organic milk and eggs come from animals not given antibiotics or hormones and fed 100% organic feed for the previous twelve months. Animals that feed on what they evolved to eat and that are given the chance to roam and forage have higher amounts of certain vitamins like A and E and more anti-inflammatory omega-3 fatty acids than their conventionally raised counterparts.[24] "Grass-fed" refers to animals raised on a ruminant (hoofed grazing mammals like cows, deer, goats, and sheep) diet of grass, rather than the corn and other grains that are typically given to feedlot animals in the United States. Good, right? Sort of. This label can also be somewhat misleading. Many animals spend the last few months of their lives on grain-based diets to help them gain weight quickly, so they might still be bulked up with steroids and antibiotics. Preferably, you should look for "grass-finished" meat, which refers to cattle raised on 100% grass and forage, after weaning from their mother, without grain or other even more questionable feed.

My go-to source for checking the toxicity of foods is the Environmental Working Group (EWG), an environmental health advocacy organization that analyzes pesticide studies and ranks contamination on forty-five of the most popular fruits and vegetables.[*] The EWG's Dirty Dozen[†] are the most chemically contaminated fruits and vegetables, so when you shop, keep this list in mind and choose organic if possible:

---

[*] Check out their complete food lists and toxicity reports at www.ewg.org.

[†] Go to: www.ewg.org/foodnews/dirty-dozen.php.

- Apples
- Celery
- Cherries
- Grapes
- Greens
- Nectarines
- Peaches
- Pears
- Peppers
- Spinach
- Strawberries
- Tomatoes

The EWG's Clean Fifteen* are fruits and vegetables that are likely to have little contamination. It's safer to go with nonorganic when selecting these items:

- Asparagus
- Avocados
- Broccoli
- Cabbage
- Cantaloupe
- Cauliflower
- Corn
- Eggplant
- Honeydew melon
- Kiwi
- Mushrooms
- Onions
- Papaya
- Peas
- Pineapple

Some fish contain mercury, a heavy metal, and other pollutants, making it unsafe to eat swordfish, shark, catfish, and tuna too often. Otherwise, fish provides us with essential, anti-inflammatory omega-3 fatty acids that our gut, brain, and vagina need to be happy. The only caveat is that harmful chemicals build up in fish fat, so trim fillets before cooking and don't eat the skin. (Sorry, salmon skin sushi lovers.)

The Environmental Defense Fund (EDF), a nonprofit organization founded in the United States in 1967 by a group of scientists, analyzes contaminants in fish. Per the EDF, the following seafood is on the list of types that are safe to eat four or more times per month[†]:

- Anchovies
- Clams
- Cod
- Crab
- Crawfish
- Haddock
- Herring
- Lobster
- Mackerel
- Mussels
- Oysters
- Salmon
- Sardines
- Scallops
- Shrimp
- Squid
- Tilapia

---

[*] Go to: www.ewg.org/foodnews/dirty-dozen.php.

[†] For more information, go to: https://seafood.edf.org/seafood-health-alerts

BLOAT BUSTERS

THE LEAST GLAMOROUS FEELING IN the world is having a bloated gut due to occasional gas, constipation, or water retention. Why does it happen? We can blame the usual suspects of sugar, gluten, dairy, red meat, toxins, hormonal imbalance, gut imbalance, too much salt, and getting your period. To zero in on the cause, my company's medical advisor Dr. Francis recommends keeping a diary to track what you ate before your swelling to learn the foods to avoid.

Other strategies to fix or prevent that pumped-up feeling are:

EAT MORE FIBER. Along with feeding gut bacteria, fiber acts like a broom in your digestive tract, sweeping up dead bacteria cells and undigested food as it moves along. 50% of women don't get enough fiber. Just by increasing fiber intake, you can move poop and gas out of your body more efficiently.

DRINK MORE WATER. Fiber is not going to move through a desert-dry gut. Picture a slip and slide. If it's dry, nothing is going to glide across it. Adding water makes it fun and slippery. Stay hydrated to flush your digestive tract and soften stool so it doesn't get stuck.

SUPPLEMENT WITH DIGESTIVE ENZYMES. If you get terrible gas when you eat dairy products, you might be deficient in the enzyme that breaks down lactose. If you blow up when you eat beans, it's possible you have a deficiency in the alpha-galactosidase, the enzyme that digests legumes. Even those without enzyme deficiencies can most likely benefit from supplements that contain amylase to break down starch, protease and pepsin to break down proteins, and lipase to break down fats.

DRINK DEBLOATING TEAS. Peppermint, chamomile, dandelion root, ginger, and fennel teas are natural diuretics that help reduce water retention, as well as support your intestinal tract. The more you drink, the less puffy you'll likely feel.

HAPPY GUT

Your gut and its microbiome work furiously hard to keep you healthy and well. Give them some love and gratitude by making a few small supportive tweaks to your life and diet:

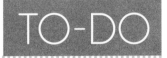

- Remember the happy gut trifecta of prebiotics + probiotics = postbiotics. Try probiotic supplements and eat vegetables, fruit, and grains to feed good bacteria and build up postbiotic gold nuggets.

- Go organic, whenever possible. You don't have to obsess about it, which could cause gut-damaging stress. To ease into it, start by buying organic eggs. Then add meats and fish. Then make the move to organic vegetables and fruits.

- Eat the rainbow: Fruits and vegetables provide us with much needed fiber. Colorful ones—red, orange, yellow, green, and purple—are rich in detoxifying phytonutrients, chlorophyll, and antioxidants that hunt down and neutralize free radicals (mutated cells that could become cancerous). Strive to eat many servings of different-colored plants per day for a happy gut.

- Always wash and peel your produce to remove residual pesticide. Check the produce aisle at your supermarket for produce washes, and choose one that is organic. Or just clean produce with a simple one-part vinegar and one-part water solution you make at home. Peeling fruit and vegetables removes pesticide residues on the skin or rind. There's not a lot you can do to wash away chemicals in fruit flesh, though.

- When you eat is just as important as what you eat. Time restricted eating—fasting on alternate days or limiting your feeding time to ten or a few hours per day—gives the gut a rest for a significant chunk of time. Mice studies have found that this practice made the gut wall stronger and lowered the number of bad gut bacteria while increasing good bacteria and postbiotic yield.[25] Just don't eat for fourteen hours a day, and your gut will thank you.

- Take pride in what you're doing for yourself. Just having the knowledge to make decisions that will keep your gut healthy is a huge first step toward whole body harmony.

chapter 7

HAPPY BRAIN

Y ou must have some serious thoughts and concerns about the functioning of your crowning GBV axis organ, chiefly: Is your brain happy?

1. My blood sugar is in the prediabetic or diabetic range. T or F

2. I drink one or more alcohol units (a beer, a glass of wine, a cocktail) per day on average. T or F

3. I would describe myself as a sedentary person. T or F

4. I feel constantly overwhelmed by the demands of life. T or F

5. My memory isn't as sharp as it used to be. I lose things, forget names, and can't remember the right words. T or F

6. I try to concentrate but laser focus eludes me. It's becoming an issue at work. T or F

7. The slightest thing can trigger a full-on stress response. T or F

8. If I'm lucky, I get six hours of sleep per night. T or F

9. I have an autoimmune disease or condition. T or F

10. I have a very cranky gut: constipation, bloating, diarrhea, cramping. T or F

11. I can't seem to shake a bad or sad mood. T or F

12. I don't remember what I ate for dinner on Monday. T or F

If you answered "True" to eight or more of the statements, you're telling me your brain is probably glum, probably leaky, and in need of intervention to turn your cognition, focus, memory, and mood around.

If you answered "False" to eight or more of the statements, congrats! Your brain is probably jolly and healthy as can be, and you'll be able to take in the fascinating science stuff coming up in this chapter without having to read the same paragraph over and over again.

Most of our brains fall somewhere between sharp and slack, and we experience occasional symptoms like fogginess, feeling stressed out, and other mood concerns. To me, the scariest aspect of leaky brain is that the damage can add up. If you have chronic brain fog when you're young, it can turn into bigger, scarier issues when you're older. Fear not! It's never too late to start taking better care of yourself, and there are a lot of ways to support brain health right now and live a happier, healthier life.

As a leaky brain is usually caused by a leaky gut, the first fix is to get your gut back in balance. For plumbing tools that can help you do that, see the previous chapter. And while you're balancing the microbiome and supporting its recovery by reducing the amount of toxins that get into the gut, there are easy simultaneous steps to support the brain, too.

Happy Brain Goal #1: Cleanup

The brain has its own dedicated cleanup operation called the glymphatic system.

How it works: The brain allows cerebrospinal fluid to flood *into* the brain, bringing essential nutrients like glucose, lipids, amino acids, and neurotransmitters with it. When the fluid rushes back out, it takes brain trash, like inflammatory molecules, toxins, and cellular waste with it. Think about it like a trash route, but the garbage collector comes into your house at night, and then dumps the trash in the yard. In this analogy, the house is your brain and the yard is your body or your lymphatic system. Weird, right? It sounds made up. But it happens inside your skull daily . . . but only while you're sleeping.

When unconscious, your brain's interstitial spaces (the gaps between cells) expand, allowing the fluid to flood powerfully into every nook and cranny to sweep up the trash and flush it out rapidly. If your brain isn't cleaned up nightly, neurotoxic trash piles up. If you've ever been sleep deprived before, you know what I mean. It's a horror show of bleak moods, fogginess, forgetfulness, and hair-trigger stress and anxiety—because your fluid couldn't sweep up the garbage effectively.

Remember it this way: No sleep, no sweep.

Not just *any* sleep activates the glymphatic system. It must be *deep* sleep. Deep (slow wave or Delta wave) sleep starts about forty-five minutes after sleep onset and is characterized by lowered heart rate and body temperature, relaxed muscles, and no rapid eye movement (REM). Most people require five ninety-minute "sleep cycles" per night. Each cycle includes two stages of light sleep, followed by two stages of deep sleep, ending with a period of REM, and then you start over with a new cycle. We spend about 20% to 30% of our total sleep time in deep sleep, with a higher per-cycle percentage during the first half of the night. The amount of time spent in each stage (light, deep, and REM) differs per person, cycle, and night. I don't want to short-change the importance of REM sleep. We need plenty of it, too, for cognitive functions like consolidating memory, learning, processing life events, and creativity.[1] The bulk of REM comes in the second half of the night, so a short sleep might be enough to clean your brain, but it's not enough to improve how well you focus, think, and remember. We need it all, really.

SYMPTOMS OF INADEQUATE DEEP SLEEP

Because you're, well, *asleep*, it's not easy to know when you haven't gotten enough deep sleep. Here are some of the symptoms that are your brain's way of saying, "I am NOT happy":

- Waking up exhausted
- Disorganized thoughts
- Fogginess
- Lack of focus
- A quick temper
- Slow reaction time
- Forgetfulness
- Sluggish immune response

"Your brain knows which stages it needs and how long to spend in each one," said Michael Breus, PhD, sleep expert and author of *Energize!* "When your body and brain have gotten what they need from each stage over a full night's rest, you'll wake up naturally feeling refreshed. For some, that might take eight hours. Others need nine, and some can get by on six or seven."

The worst-case scenario for sleep quality is skidding along the surface of light sleep for too long and never plunging into the deep, brain-sweeping stage of the cycle. A few factors cause this particularly devious sleep disruption: the blue light from phones, alcohol within a couple of hours of bedtime, caffeine within several hours of bedtime, a partner who tosses and turns, sleep medications, recreational drugs, and a too-hot room. If you drink a glass of wine to help you fall asleep, it's no wonder that you wake up tired and foggy. (Not that I have any personal experience with that . . . okay, not *much*.)

My friend whose brain fog was so severe she had to take a leave of absence from her tech job, had been taking zolpidem, a prescription sleeping pill, for months at a time. Research shows that, although zolpidem might help you fall asleep (not much more than a placebo, though) and doesn't impact REM sleep, it does interfere with getting quality deep sleep[2] that the brain needs to take out the trash. When she figured that out, she started to taper off her meds until she could sleep naturally—and she added probiotics!

Sleep drugs can act as microbiome disruptors, too, which is another reason to try to cut down or cut them out. If you want to get off zolpidem or any other sleep drug (OTC or prescription), do not go cold turkey. Taper off incrementally, like she did, under the supervision of a doctor.

To ensure higher quality sleep, Dr. Breus recommends sleep hygiene practices that train the brain to fall asleep quickly, stay down, and wake up clear and energized. They work for severe insomnia patients, so they might work for you.

- WAKE UP **at the same time each day.**

- GO TO SLEEP **at the same time each night.**

- NO CAFFEINE **after 3:00 pm.**

- NO ALCOHOL **within a few hours of bedtime.**

- SHUT DOWN. **Blue light from devices suppresses the release of melatonin, the sleep hormone. An hour before bedtime, turn them off. Maybe even put them in a different room. A recent study of 1,500 Americans found that 90% used devices within an hour of bedtime. Researchers compared the impact of before-bed reading of a printed book to an e-reader. The people using e-readers were less sleepy at bedtime, had a harder time falling asleep, had reduced melatonin secretion, and felt less awake in the morning.[3] If you must use a device before bed, use blue-light screen blockers or glasses.**

- DECELERATE. During the off-screen hour before bed, slow down your thoughts and try to relax by meditating, journaling, reading a print book, and stretching, or taking a hot bath, using only pH balancing soaps and salts, of course. Dr. Breus recommends doing a calming breath technique that quiets the adrenals (the glands that release cortisol and adrenaline) and stimulates the vagus nerve: inhale through the nose and into the belly for a count of four; hold the breath for a count of seven; exhale through the mouth for a count of eight. Repeat as necessary.

- PREPARE THE ROOM. Make your bedroom the ideal sleep environment. Lower the thermostat to 65 degrees, use blackout curtains or an eye mask to block light, and turn on white noise or use ear plugs to block sound.

- SLEEP SOLO. If your partner keeps you up, relocate to the couch. Or send them there.

EXTREME SLEEP ISSUES

THERE IS NO BRAIN HAPPINESS without getting enough deep sleep. If good sleep hygiene practices don't get you there on your own, you might have a sleep disorder. If you suspect that you do, talk to your primary care doctor and get a referral to a sleep specialist or seek info at the sleep center finder portal at the American Academy of Sleep Medicine.[*] Insomnia and sleep apnea are no joke. Telltale signs are taking an hour or more to fall asleep, waking up throughout the night, not being able to fall back to sleep, loud snoring and breathing interruptions. If left untreated, sleep disorders can rob you of brain cleaning time and might cause serious cognitive and mood conditions. Most insurance providers will cover treatment.

---

[*] Go to: sleepeducation.org/sleep-center/.

LOVE YOURSELF WELL

Happy Brain Goal #2: Tamp Down

The glymphatic system does a five-star job of keeping your brain clean, if you get enough sleep and—this is key—your gut is healthy. To give your brain's cleanup crew a fighting chance, tamp down on what may be impacting your brain and mental health as much as possible.

Basically, if your gut is leaky, trouble will continue to trickle upstream into the brain. During my rough year, with my vitamin deficiency, ravaged-by-antibiotics microbiome, and leaky gut, I would sleep for ten hours a night—and even that wasn't enough. See the following sections for some advice on supporting gut and brain health and giving the cleanup crew a clear path in your brain!

ANTI-PUFF DIET

Anti-inflammatory foods—those that feed your brain with protein and essential vitamins and minerals—are also *anti*oxidants. I'd heard that word a million times before I understood what it meant. To explain what antioxidants are and what they can do, I have to back up and talk about oxidation first.

Oxidation means something is exposed to oxygen, to air. When a sliced apple or a halved avocado is exposed to oxygen, the flesh turns brown. When metal is oxidated, it rusts. This means the item is aging and degrading earlier than it normally would because of the exposure. But there's more to it than that! When this corrosion happens to your inner organs, it's sometimes referred to as "oxidative stress." When oxidative stress gets out of hand, it can cause rapid aging of your cells, and negatively impact health.

How do you keep it in check?

Well, that brings us back to the beginning of this section. The brain requires a lot of oxygen to function—20% of our body's supply. All that oxygen exposure produces a lot of free radicals (rough cells) up there, making the brain particularly vulnerable to oxidative stress.

To sum it up: Oxidation: bad. Oxidative stress: horrible. Free radicals: mostly evil.

The saviors in this story, and the heroes of cranial joy, are antioxidants. Their glory is in the name. They work *against* (anti) agents of corrosion (oxidants) that harm us.

Antioxidants—like vitamins A, C, and E, carotenoids, selenium, manganese, lycopene, flavonoids, and hundreds of other substances—neutralize free radicals. They fix their mutation and render them completely inert. And since free radicals and stress in the brain can be so potentially dangerous, eating an antioxidant-rich diet is essential for brain happiness.

GIVE YOUR BRAIN SOME LOVE WITH ANTIOXIDANTS

Slow aging and stave off neurodegeneration with these anti-puff options:

- Artichokes
- Asparagus
- Avocados
- Beans
- Beets
- Blueberries
- Broccoli
- Carrots

- Cherries
- Dark chocolate
- Green tea
- Kale
- Mushrooms
- Olive oil
- Peppers
- Potatoes

- Pumpkin
- Raspberries
- Red cabbage
- Spinach
- Squash
- Strawberries
- Sweet potatoes
- Tomatoes

Add antioxidants into your meals by literally sprinkling them on your food. Spices like cayenne, black pepper, ginger, and garlic have anti-inflammatory compounds. Curcumin (a substance found in turmeric, an orange/yellow spice) has been shown to bond with toxic heavy metals like lead. In effect, curcumin grabs hold of the metals and drags them out of the body, potentially reducing neurotoxicity and tissue damage.[4] Grate fresh turmeric root, boil it in filtered water and drink it as a tea, or add ground turmeric in anything for more color, flavor, and anti-puff powers to food.

Foods that may cause inflammation are to be avoided whenever possible. (I know it's not easy!) You already know what they are: refined carbohydrates like white bread, crackers, and pastries, fried food, added sugars, alcohol, red meat, processed meat (any protein that comes in a tube or a strip), as well as saturated fat in margarine, shortening, and lard. As much as you can, avoid the siren call of fast food chains.

SOOTHING EXERCISE

Physical activity can have a detoxifying effect on the brain. We all know this to be true intuitively—"I'm going to take a walk to clear my head"— but the mechanisms of how this works are not completely understood. There is evidence that regular exercise can help:

- Diminish blood-brain barrier (BBB) leaks by increasing the density of the epithelial cells in its capillaries

- Make antioxidants even better at neutralizing free radicals, thereby reducing oxidative stress[5]

- Boost blood flow to the brain that supports cell growth

- Support mental clarity

- Enhance sleep quality[6]

- Support glymphatic functioning[7]

Recent research has found that combining exercise with an antioxidant and omega-3 fatty acid–rich diet compounds the health-supporting effects in the brain.[8] If you had a nice meal of wild-caught salmon, a spinach salad, and a bowl of yogurt and berries for dessert, and then took an after-dinner walk with a friend, you might just generate brain cell growth (a process called neurogenesis), improve vascular function, and feel better about your whole life.

But how much exercise are we talking about? Good news, actually: You don't have to pick up kickboxing. Thirty minutes a day of stretching or walking will work just fine. You don't even have to do them all at once. It's cumulative; ten minutes here, five there, just get to thirty. During the back-to-normal process, it's preferable not to go ham on HIIT (high-intensity interval training) at the gym. Strenuous exercise elevates cortisol, a known culprit of degrading the GALT, jamming the vagus nerve, and unsealing GBV axis leaks. Instead, stick to stretching, strolling, dancing, and sex to trigger the release of energizing endorphins and calming serotonin, hormones that make your brain, and you, happy. And while you're having fun and increasing blood flow, you're de-stressing and stimulating new brain cell growth.

WARNING: BRAIN DETOX SIDE EFFECTS

As you clean and calm the brain, it doesn't get happy right away. It might even feel grumpy for up to a week. Detox isn't always fun. The side effects are worth it, though, once you get to the other side. Some common reactions to brain detox include headaches, irritability, muscle ache, nausea, cravings, fatigue, and poor sleep.

BRAIN TRAINING

SCIENTISTS ONCE THOUGHT THE BRAIN stopped developing after the first few years of life. But new research has shown that the brain can form new neural pathways and reshape itself in response to behavioral repetition. The science of how the brain can reshape and rewire itself is called neuroplasticity. By sleeping enough, exercising, and eating well habitually, you can train your brain to make healthy, happy choices automatically. And as your brain rewires for health and happiness, it prunes away old, bad habits, so they become less and less appealing.

To promote new brain cell growth and blaze new happy neural pathways:

TRAVEL. Traveling promotes neurogenesis by exposing your brain to new and complex environments. Just taking a weekend road trip to a different city stimulates your brain.

PLAY A GAME. Memory games promote connection in your brain's prefrontal parietal network and can slow memory loss with age.

PLAY AN INSTRUMENT. Brain scans on musicians show heightened connectivity between brain regions. The intense, multisensory experience of combining motor actions with specific sounds leads to the formation of new neural networks.

SWITCH SIDES. Try brushing your teeth or stirring your tea with your nondominant hand. The simple switch strengthens connectivity between your brain cells.

MAKE SOMETHING. It'll strengthen the neural pathways that control attention and focus.

DANCE. Free-style dancing that isn't memory dependent increases neuroplasticity because it forces you to integrate several brain functions at once: kinesthetic, rational, musical, and emotional. It's all stimulating, and that makes the brain happy.

HAPPY BRAIN

The smartest things you can do for your brain:

- Get some quality sleep. Your brain's trash-removing glymphatic system only operates when you're unconscious.

- Sleep posture affects how well the brain's waste removal system works. A study used MRI machines to compare glymphatic system efficiency when the participants were lying on their back, side, or belly. The best position for brain cleanup was lying on their side. Back sleepers did okay, too. The worst position was lying on their belly.[9] Stomach sleepers: Try rolling onto your back or side. Your brain will be happier if you do.

- Eat anti-inflammatory, antioxidant foods (rainbow-colored fruits and vegetables and spices) to neutralize the free radicals that would otherwise rust your brain.

- Help your brain with gentle exercise, ideally in combination with an antioxidant diet.

- Stimulate new brain cell growth by seeing and doing new things. The more you push your brain to expand, the healthier and happier it'll be.

TO-DO

LOVE YOURSELF WELL

chapter 8

HAPPY VAGINA

Now it's time to go deep, to get to the seat of the issue, the very core of your overall health and well-being. How's your vagina doing?

1. My vagina is itchy and hot. When in public, I squirm in my chair for relief and hope no one notices. T or F

2. I've had two or more vaginal infections in the last six months. T or F

3. My vagina is desert dry, and the skin down there is easily irritated. T or F

4. When I laugh hard, I pee myself. T or F

5. I have a cranky gut. T or F

6. I've had two or more UTIs in the last six months. T or F

7. My chronic vaginal infections are so frustrating, it seems like I have no control over my body. T or F

8. I'm so self-conscious about how I smell that I don't like doing certain sex acts. T or F

9. I always use scented soaps on my privates. T or F

10. It hurts to have vaginal penetrative intercourse. T or F

11. I'm prone to catching sexually transmitted infections. T or F

12. I haven't had an orgasm in at least a week. T or F

If you answered "True" to *any* of the statements, your vagina probably isn't nearly as happy as it deserves to be, which can lead to an unhappy you. Dr. Horton calls the vagina "the forgotten organ" because of how little consideration it gets from the medical establishment. From the human perspective, it's impossible to forget about her, even for a minute, when it's unhappy with uncomfortable symptoms.

When I had those rolling vaginal health issues, my thoughts were never far from the literal seat of my problem. I was constantly assessing what was going on down there, relief between treatments was tempered by dread that it would happen again. And when it did, I'd feel crushed and helpless and go through a grieving process over the loss. Vaginal imbalance took my peace of mind, sex life, and joy.

Getting back my vaginal happiness transformed my life, day to day, moment by moment. A big part of my mission as founder of my company is to encourage women to overcome embarrassment, take their personal health care seriously, and stop hoping that things will just get better on their own. They won't. You have to take care of your vagina so it takes care of you.

You are sitting on a source of tremendous joy. When your vagina is thriving, everything is right with the world. To glide inside, set out to realize happy vagina goals.

Happy Vagina Goal #1: Balance

Leaky vagina can be caused by an imbalance in that area's microbiome, but it often starts with gut dysbiosis. As you know, these two microbiomes have a close relationship. Whatever is going on in one microbiome, good or bad, leaks into the others. If the gut has an overgrowth of *candida*, the vagina's environment will sync up. Therefore, to rebalance the vagina, you have to start by rebalancing the gut. (See Chapter 6 for the complete rundown on that.)

THE RIGHT STRAIN

Gut probiotics can help reinforce good bacteria populations in the digestive tract, which can benefit the vagina's microbiome, too. But don't stop there. Although the two microbiomes are similar, they are not the same. To support beneficial bacteria downstairs, try a probiotic supplement that contains several strains of the dominant vagina bacteria, *Lactobacilli*.

Look for these strains in particular: *Lactobacillus acidophilus, Lactobacillus plantarum, Lactobacillus salivarius, Lactobacillus casei, Lactobacillus paracasei, Lactobacillus rhamnosus, Lactobacillus brevis*, and *Lactobacillus gasseri*. If your female-friendly probiotic supplements contain prebiotic fiber like inulin, so much the better. Or just eat more inulin in food sources like roots (chicory, yacon), bulbs (garlic, onions, shallots, leeks), and grains (rye, wheat).

Happy Vagina Goal #2: Support

By support, I mean don't make it harder for your vagina to be happy. Don't throw hazards at it. Give it the equipment and attention it needs to maintain a healthy balance, and continue to treat it right.

NO PANTIES IN A BUNCH

Rethink thongs. Reconsider G-strings, too, and any other kind of panty with a band of fabric that nestles between the butt cheeks. Bad bacteria from the anus will jump onto that fabric and march right across it, into the vagina and urethra.

I'll grant you, thongs and G-strings are justifiably popular. They have saved us all from the blight of panty lines. They feel sexy and look good. I completely get it, you would not believe how much. But wearing thongs is like playing a high-stakes game of "Would You Rather?" Is the pleasure of wearing thongs worth the heightened risk of recurrent UTIs and vaginal infections? Would you rather feel a bit dowdy in cotton briefs . . . or pee fire?

Wearing the same panties two days in a row doubles the number of bacteria in the gusset that might find their way into your vagina, urethra, and bladder. For that reason alone, change your panties daily! A friend of mine was on a cross-country camping trip and ran out of clean drawers. "I knew that wearing dirty panties increased the risk of yeast infection and UTIs, so I thought, *I'll go commando until I can wash everything*," she said. Nothing came between her and her Levi's for three days . . . and on day four, she felt the burn. "Turns out the UTI was caused by the bacteria that accumulated in the crotch of my jeans," she said.

Fabric choice matters. Choose breathable, moisture-wicking cotton or bamboo. Typically, silk, satin, or polyester is going to retain moisture, and that increases the risk of fungal skin infection. If non-cotton panties have an all-cotton gusset, though, they should be okay.

It's a controversial subject, but there is some research that says even if panties are machine washed, over time, they can still harbor bacteria. If you are so inclined, it might be a good idea to replace old undies every year or two. Places like Target have a great—affordable and cute—selection of underwear.

KEEP IT CLEAN

The vulva has a high concentration of sweat glands, hair follicles, and blood vessels, making it one of the most permeable areas of the body. Whatever you put on it is going to soak in and leak into your bloodstream. Parabens, surfactants, and phthalates are pH-disrupting chemicals that should not get within ten feet of your vulva. Check the label before buying any cleanser, wipe, foam, lotion, or gel for this area, and make sure none of those chemicals are on the ingredients list. If you don't want to use a cleaner, all you really need to clean your vulva and perineum is nature's cleanser: water.

The impulse to use scented products is based in shame. Your parts do not need to smell like lavender or passionfruit to be "fresh." A healthy, sexy vagina smells like you, like the spicy, earthy, salty woman you are. I asked a thirty-two-year-old hetero male friend about this, and he said, "Women seem to think that men are turned off by vaginal odor, and it is just not true. My theory is that in their past, women were shamed by their teenage boyfriends who were completely mystified by the vagina and confused by the smell. I promise you, grown-ass men are not afraid or turned off by the smell of a healthy vagina. *We like it.* The scent activates the lizard brain. It's instinctually and instantly arousing. When I get up close and personal with a vagina and it smells and tastes like a grapefruit, I think about dish soap. Not sexy, at all." That said, it comes down to *your* own personal preference. So if you like using feminine hygiene products, consider a fragrance-free pH-balancing cleanser with organic, gentle plant-based ingredients like aloe and calendula.

PERIOD STUFF

A typical menstrual cycle occurs every twenty-one to thirty-five days with bleeding that lasts two to seven days. However, up to 20% of women have atypical or irregular periods. Either their periods stop happening, they spot between periods, have unusually heavy bleeding, or severe pain and cramping with nausea and sometimes diarrhea. All of these symptoms might be caused by anything from use of birth control pills, to fibroids, hormonal imbalance, stress, inflammation, or a serious disease like endometriosis. If your period was as regular as clockwork, and then suddenly changed, take it seriously and visit a gynecologist.

Having a typical cycle doesn't make it any more fun. Every month, hormones and bacteria populations change and make you more vulnerable to infection. Basic period hygiene can help you avoid most of the risks.

- RINSE TWICE A DAY. **Blood can create the right environment for bad bacteria to overgrow. Wash your vulva in the morning and again at night or use an unscented pH-balancing wipe. *Do not wash inside the vagina!* Let it do its job and clean itself.**

- FOLLOW THE RULE OF FOUR. **Whether you use tampons or pads (unscented and organic ones are preferable), change them every four hours, even if they're not saturated. Leaving tampons in for too long increases the likelihood of an infection. Overnight, you can go eight hours, but no longer. Moist, sweaty pads can increase the chance of fungal infections. You are probably okay to wear a pad overnight, though, because you'll sweat less while sleeping than you would during daytime activity. (But always read the instructions that come with your tampons or pads to be sure you're using them for the appropriate amount of time.)**

- WASH YOUR HANDS BEFORE AND AFTER. **Your hands can transfer all kinds of pathogenic bacteria to the area when inserting or removing tampons and pads.**

WHAT ABOUT CRAMPS?

The hormonal shifts make you vulnerable to just feeling lousy. Dr. Horton has some bio-hacks that can help get you through a bad week and not let your period get the better of you:

- **ESSENTIAL OILS.** Organic essential oils made from rose, lavender, sage, or geranium can be mixed with organic carrier oils like coconut or avocado and massaged into your lower abdomen to reduce cramps, inflammation, and bloating. To be most effective, start rubbing the week before your period begins.

- **SUPPLEMENTS.** Be extra vigilant about taking fiber supplements, multivitamins with calcium, magnesium, iron, and vitamins E, B6, B12, and omega-3s during your period to get you through the hard times.

- **HEAT.** "Heat therapy is an easy and effective way to reduce cramps or lower back pain associated with menstruation," she said. So break out a heating pad and press it directly on your back or front to help your muscles unclench.

- **TEA.** Put on your lounge pants, get snuggly on the couch with a blanket, and have a cup of tea. "Ginger tea is rich in anti-inflammatory and pain-relieving properties," said Dr. Horton. "Chamomile tea will help soothe you to sleep and has anti-inflammatory and anti-spasmodic properties to help alleviate menstrual cramps. Cinnamon tea is a powerful antioxidant that helps reduce inflammation and bloating associated with menstruation."

MENSTRUAL CUPS

By using menstrual cups—popular brands are DivaCup, Cora, and MeLuna—you will save money *and* the planet. A lifetime of tampons costs approximately $2,000. A menstrual cup costs around $25 and can be used for ten years, making the total cost for four decades of menstruating around only $100. Rubber or silicone menstrual cups aren't recyclable. But they are a lot more sustainable than the millions of single-use tampons and pads that wind up in landfills, sewers, and the ocean each year.

But are cups safe? According to an international meta-review of forty-three studies and thousands of participants, menstrual cups are safe and effective tools for menstrual management.[1] The risk of toxic shock syndrome, which is caused by an overgrowth of the bacteria *Staphylococcus aureus*, is slightly greater compared to tampons, but still quite rare.[2]

Putting anything into the vagina holds some risk of infection, be it a tampon, menstrual cup, sex toy, or penis. As long as you insert the cup with clean hands, sanitize it every twelve hours (using nonscented, oil-free pH-balancing soap), boil it between uses, and store it in a breathable fabric pouch, it's unlikely to cause infection. Fit and placement are important. If the cup is too wide for your body or improperly positioned, it can push through the vaginal wall into the urethra, impeding urine flow and possibly causing a UTI. Ask your ob/gyn for recommendations and advice on brands and fit, or just go back to nonscented tampons.

WORK THE PELVIC FLOOR

The ultimate vaginal support is the pelvic floor, which is a hammock of muscles that slings from the pubic bone in front to the coccyx (tail bone) in back. It holds the pelvic organs—the bladder, uterus, vagina, and rectum—in place.

Dr. Desai is a urogynecologist who specializes in pelvic floor disorders, like prolapses (when muscles and ligaments are so weak that body parts fall out), and incontinence (loss of control that allows urine and feces to escape unintentionally). "Childbirth tends to be one of the highest risks for prolapse and incontinence," said Dr. Desai. "I see women post-delivery who are suddenly peeing themselves. But there are other risk factors, like genetics and age."

Women in their twenties, thirties, and forties can start now to be mindful of their pelvic floor so that, later, their parts stay inside where they belong. "There's so many little things that you can do every day to incorporate protection to the pelvic floor," said Dr. Desai. It's not a guarantee that you'll never have any issues, unfortunately, but lifting with the legs, using glute and quadricep muscles to stand up or get out of the car, strengthening your core, and decreasing intra-abdominal pressure (the bearing-down feeling when you cough or poop) are only going to help.

"Everyone knows about Kegels, contracting muscles to tone the pelvic floor, but you have to do them the right way," warned Dr. Desai. "What I see often in exams is that people *think* they're Kegeling, but really, they're just pushing." By flexing the wrong muscles, women can end up tightening their pelvic floor in a way that makes it *really* difficult to unclench. Per Dr. Desai, you can unlearn wrong-way Kegel flexing, and relearn to do them the right way.

FIRST RELAX. Lie on your back with your knees bent and feet resting comfortably on the floor. Do a few deep belly breaths to relax your abdomen and back.

ISOLATE THE RIGHT MUSCLES. Imagine a straw inside your vagina. (Don't put one in; just visualize it.) Tighten the vaginal muscles around the straw and then release. Practice holding and letting go several times to isolate which muscles to contract. Caution: Don't lift the hips or tense your abs. Keep the body *relaxed*. The only muscles that move should be within the vagina.

BUILD ENDURANCE. Work up to holding each contraction for ten seconds before relaxing. Eventually, your muscles will become stronger, and you'll be able to hold for fifteen to twenty seconds at a time.

REPEAT. The pelvic floor muscles are like any other. You have to put in the effort to see results. Perform sets of ten Kegels, three times per day, several days per week. After three months, you'll see an improvement.

The pelvic floor and the core muscles are interrelated, both providing stability and support throughout the back and hips. If you work on your core, you're also strengthening the pelvic floor. Here are a couple combos that exercise both simultaneously:

GLUTE BRIDGE. Lie on your back with both feet on the floor and your knees bent. Gently raise your pelvis toward the sky while contracting the glutes *and* doing a Kegel. Hold the pose for five seconds and then lower your hips to the floor.

SUPERMAN. Lie flat on your stomach with your arms and legs outstretched. Slowly raise your arms, shoulders, and legs off the ground while contracting your back muscles and glutes, and then throw a Kegel in the mix, too. Hold for five seconds and release.

One last thing: Like clenching the jaw or tensing the shoulders, we flex our pelvic floor when we're under stress. We don't even realize how much tension we carry in our inner hammocks. When in stressful situations, check in with your pelvic floor and mindfully relax it. Do the same for your jaw and shoulders while you're at it.

VAGINAL PHYSICAL THERAPY: IT'S A THING

Back in her twenties, a friend of mine started to experience painful sex. She had the desire, but it hurt too much. Needless to say, this didn't help her relationship.

She went to her gynecologist, who said, "Your pelvic floor is just really tight. You need to go to a vaginal physical therapist."

"A *what*?" she thought. "Who knew there were private practitioners out there, beyond a traditional ob/gyn, who could help with this very specific problem? I sure didn't. If I hadn't been referred to a VPT by my doctor, it's possible I never would have been able to enjoy penetrative sex again," she told me.

At vagina therapy, she relearned to relax. "My boyfriend and I could have sex again and it didn't hurt anymore, which was the highest praise I could give this therapy," she said.

"I send 75% of my patients to pelvic floor/vaginal physical therapy," said Dr. Desai. Most of her patients had no idea such practitioners existed.

A session takes place in a private room, where the licensed therapist (who's had years of training) does an external and an internal exam. The external exam is an assessment of core muscles. For the internal exam, the therapist inserts a finger into the patient's vagina to assess the pelvic floor muscles from the inside.

Depending on the symptoms, the therapist will prescribe specific exercises. For example, stress incontinence due to advanced age or childbirth is caused by a lack of pelvic floor support around the urethra. The therapist will work with the patient to contract specific muscles to increase strength around it. When the patient sneezes, she knows to flex the appropriate muscles to prevent an accident.

Over the coming decade, Dr. Desai predicts that VPT will go mainstream. "After delivering a child vaginally, every woman should have pelvic floor physical therapy for three to six months as a baseline," she said. "Peeing yourself doesn't have to become the new normal for new moms. Although many just accept it and wait for years with symptoms before they see a urogynecologist like me. In the meantime, they spend a fortune on pads. They're exhausted. They leak during intercourse. It takes an emotional toll."

Like so many other conditions, pelvic floor disorders have become something women think they just have to live with on their own. Maybe they don't look for help because of the embarrassment factor. Relief from symptoms is so much greater than the momentary shame of admitting to someone that you have them. You can be cured, if you advocate for yourself and find a skilled, licensed professional to help.[*]

---

[*] Go to https://pelvicrehab.com/ to find a board certified VPT practitioner near you.

Happy Vagina Goal #3: Intimacy

Love your sexy self by getting to know your vagina, intimately.

TAKE A LOOK

Vulva mapping is like a self-guided exploration of every cranny, fold, and nub of your genitals. (For a refresher on your genital parts, go to page 33.) It should only take about ten minutes to identify the vital parts, from the clitoris at the top to the anus at the bottom, and all the openings, lips, and sensitive bits in between. Make a drawing, if so inspired. How can you love something that you've never even looked at? It's not scary! It's beautiful because it's a very important part of you.

"Many, many patients tell me that they don't like how they look because one of their labia minora is longer than the other," said Dr. Horton. "How you feel about your appearance matters. It can affect your self-esteem and your desire to be sexual." She suspects the concern about symmetry started from early exposure to porn or a remark from an ignorant boyfriend. "Criticism early on in their sexual lives makes women self-conscious," she said. "Could you imagine if a girl told her boyfriend, 'Wow, your dick is really small!' How often would that happen? Girls are worried that boys will like them and that they look 'normal.' Every day, women ask me about labiaplasty, a surgical procedure to trim their inner lips. I tell them, 'No one is symmetrical. You are normal and fine.'"

DON'T *JUST* LOOK

Touch yourself, as if you are doing it for the very first time (or for the first time). By slowly examining, inch by inch, the vulva you've just mapped, you will make new discoveries of erogenous zones you didn't know you had. Go slow, stay curious. Vary your touch, from feathery stroking, gentle scratching, tapping, pressing, vibrating with a toy.

During orgasm, your brain releases serotonin, oxytocin, and endorphins that make you feel happy, loving, and content. The more oxytocin and serotonin you have, the less cortisol and stress. Endorphins decrease anxiety and improve sleep. Better sleep boosts brain detox and energy. When you have an orgasm and release the happy hormones, you'll automatically switch into "safe and social" parasympathetic nervous system mode. Not only is it physically possible to have a VN-stimulation orgasm, having an orgasm stimulates the VN. Another win-win.

Dr. Horton prescribes masturbating regularly as a treatment for sexual dysfunction, female orgasmic disorder, and just feeling better about everything. It's a readily accessible form of recreation that raises levels of happy hormones like oxytocin, serotonin, dopamine, and adrenaline, all of which boost self-esteem and can even make you feel more optimistic and purposeful about your life.[3] Some might fear that masturbation somehow takes away from sexual pleasure with a partner. If anything, it puts sex top of mind. When you think about pleasure, you want more of it. Heightened desire and intimate self-knowledge makes sex with a partner more satisfying for both of you.

For those who are masturbation pros, carry on doing what you do. For those who don't have a masturbation practice, it's time to get to know your body and what makes you feel good.

An excellent place to start is the clitoris. The part you can see on the outside is called the glans, that pea-sized button at the top of the vulva, hiding under a chic little hood of skin. When aroused, the glans becomes erect and peeks out from under the hood, making it easier to find when you're turned on. The glans has 8,000 nerve endings. By comparison, the penis has 4,000. (The clitoris wins.)

The glans is just the tip of the iceberg. Most of the whole clitoral body is below the surface. It's got legs called crura that extend into the pelvis on either side of the pubic bone, and teardrop-shaped three-and-a-half-inch-long vestibule bulbs. The crura and vestibule bulbs have erectile tissue, too. They swell when aroused, which triggers an increase of lubrication via two glands in the vagina. The Bartholin's glands secrete acidic mucus, and the Skene's glands, located on each side of the urethra, secrete lubricating fluid into the urethra and the vagina. Skene's glands also produce a milky white discharge during sexual arousal comprised of enzymes and proteins that is called "female ejaculate." If you haven't noticed it, no big deal. The substance doesn't make orgasms better. It's just a cool thing we can do.

"There's still a taboo and a lot of shame about touching yourself," said Dr. Horton. "Masturbation and self-exploration are among the best ways to erase the shame around your body and undo negative messaging that you might have received." It's not your fault if you're squeamish about your vagina. But it's your responsibility to push through shame blocks, to know and love your vagina so it'll love you back.

GIVE YOUR LANDING STRIP SOME LOVE

Shaving pubic hair goes in and out of fashion. It's a personal decision, but if you are a fan or a first-time trimmer, Dr. Horton would like you to follow a few safety rules:

- Warm the area first. Shave after a bath or shower to make the hair softer and easier to shave.

- Use shaving cream or gel to protect your skin.

- Use a fresh blade, not the dull razor that's been sitting in your shower caddy for a year.

- Shave along the grain to avoid nicks.

- Exfoliate gently in the shower to prevent ingrown hairs, bumps, and cysts.

- If you do get a cyst, use a warm compress to open it up. Then cover it with antibiotic gel and a bandage.

BIRTH CONTROL

To be intimate with a male partner, you will probably use some form of birth control. As mentioned earlier, condoms with spermicide can potentially kill the beneficial bacteria in the vagina and tip the pH into dangerous alkalinity. (So can sperm, by the way.) If you are among the approximately 9% of women whose number one choice of contraception is condoms, you should consider trying spermicide-free, fragrance-free, water-soluble, and silicone-based lubes.

As for the approximately 26%[4] of women who are using the pill, an implant, a Depo-Provera shot, a ring, an IUD, or a patch, be advised that hormonal birth control methods may make you more susceptible to leaky gut, recurrent yeast infections,[5] inflammatory bowel diseases,[6] and lowered microbiome diversity. It's all about weighing the benefits and the risks. If hormonal contraception works for you and hasn't caused you any leaky gut or vaginal problems, it's probably fine to continue using it. But if you have recurrent infections and gut issues, your birth control method might be contributing to your pain and suffering.

Dr. Francis explains the potential effects of birth control pills on the gut microbiome: Certain species in the microbiome have the important job of metabolizing (breaking down) excess estrogen in the body and getting rid of used estrogen. When you take birth control pills, you can create a double-barreled problem, by increasing estrogen levels while simultaneously decreasing the specific types of bacteria that metabolize it.[7] If we can't round up and break down excess estrogen, we're stuck with it. It gets reabsorbed into our tissues, causing a condition called "estrogen dominance." "Right now, we have a lot of problems in our culture with this type of hormone imbalance," said Dr. Francis. Low-grade symptoms may include bloating, irregular periods, mood swings, weight gain, hair loss, anxiety, breast tenderness. It can get much more serious. "Estrogen dominance causes fibroid cysts, endometriosis, and breast cancer," she said.

Happy Vagina Goal #4: Treat

For a bacterial or yeast overgrowth, boric acid suppositories can work well. But you should always consult your health care practicitioner for your best options. Often, Dr. Horton prescribes oral antibiotics like metronidazole or clindamycin gel.

Trust me, any overgrowth that's left untreated will get worse. If you suspect you're dealing with a UTI—there is no mistaking the burn and the urge to go every five seconds—go to your doctor or an urgent care facility, have your urine tested, and get treated with antibiotics. You should also ask about taking probiotics to maintain good bacteria populations during and after a course of antibiotics. Perimenopausal, menopausal, and postmenopausal women who have decreased estrogen levels and chronic UTIs are having great success with prescription vaginal estrogen cream treatment.

The best thing for overall vaginal and urinary tract health, though, is taking care of your own body and being mindful about good practices.

E. coli can often travel from the anus to the urethra. To avoid helping that along, whether you're peeing or pooping, wipe front to back. Never, ever, ever, under fear of God, wipe from the anus in the direction of the vagina or urethra, or from the vagina toward the urethra!

As daily probiotics maintain acidic vulvovaginal pH, supplements can help support your urinary tract. Other preventative supplement options are:

- **PROANTHOCYANIDIN (PAC), a cranberry fruit extract clinically proven to support urinary tract health.**[8]

- **D-MANNOSE, a simple sugar that hinders bacteria from sticking to urinary tract walls and has been shown to be an effective treatment and prophylactic agent.**[9]

- **VITAMIN D, our dear friend, can help to support urinary and vaginal health.**

During sex, bacteria is easily transferred from one part to the other. But, if you pee afterwards, the flow of urine carries the harmful bacteria out of the urethra and into the toilet where it can't do you any harm. In fact, the more water you drink, the more you pee, the better chance you have of dislodging any bacteria from sticking to your bladder. So, drink eight glasses of water per day and don't hold it in. If you feel the urge to pee, do it. Otherwise, you're giving bacteria in your urinary tract the opportunity to grow.

SEXUALLY TRANSMITTED INFECTIONS

Another good thing about condoms is that they prevent STIs, which are harder and harder to avoid. According to the Centers for Disease Control, every year, there are 20 million new cases of STIs in the United States. If you're sexually active or in a new relationship, get tested for HIV, herpes, gonorrhea, chlamydia, hepatitis, and syphilis. Even if you haven't had too much action recently, screening for STIs should be part of your annual check-up, just to be sure. Chlamydia and gonorrhea testing is just a vaginal swab, no big deal. To rule out HIV, hepatitis, and syphilis, you'll have to give some blood, a small sacrifice for peace of mind. The detection of herpes (a virus that one in five Americans carry) and genital warts (from the human papillomavirus, the most common STI) is done the old-fashioned way, by looking for sores and bumps, and possibly, a swab for the lab. Some STIs have no symptoms, though, so regular testing is helpful!

If you test positive, it does not mean you are dirty or morally corrupt. You caught a virus or a bug, and now that you have that knowledge, you can deal with it. People used to die from STIs that we can cure easily today, so at least be happy that we have the tools to heal. What comes next might not be so joyous, having "the talk" with a sexual partner (or a few) about your diagnosis, whether they gave it to you, or you gave it to them, and what it means for the relationship. Regardless, use a condom until you're both treated and cured.

SPECIAL CIRCUMSTANCES

During certain times of life, your vagina might need extra care to be happy.

IF YOU'RE TRYING TO GET PREGNANT...

- REDUCE STRESS. It might be a challenge, because trying to get pregnant can be stressful. As you know, stress means cortisol flooding, and cortisol tips the pH balance in the vagina toward alkaline. Practice breathing techniques, meditation, and gentle movement to maintain normal cortisol levels and keep pH on point.

- CHECK YOUR PH. If you are taking high doses of hormones during an in vitro fertilization (IVF) cycle, your vaginal pH is going to shift from acidic to alkaline, which can put you at a higher risk for vaginal imbalance. Taking probiotics can keep you in balance.

IF YOU'RE PREGNANT...

- DON'T PANIC. Things are going to change every single day, with increased blood flow, hormonal shifts, ligaments stretching, and increased pressure in the area. Changes in discharge and scent are to be expected and are usually not a cause of concern. New experience brings new feelings. Just be mindful of what's happening so you can discuss the changes with your ob/gyn at your next appointment. If you have intense pain and bleeding, call your doctor immediately.

- PROTECT THE AREA. You don't have to put yellow police tape across your vulva. But be vigilant about not introducing any bacteria that shouldn't be in there. Consider using pH-balancing soap and lube on your parts. Sex is fine, unless your ob/gyn has said otherwise.

- STOP KEGELING. If you overdo it, hypertonic muscles can prevent you from being able to relax enough to push effectively or allow the baby's head to come through the birth canal. With doctor approval, do Kegels the right way (see instructions earlier in this chapter).

- GET CHECKED FOR UTIS. Pregnant women are much more susceptible to becoming gravely ill from a UTI, and this can increase the risk of preterm delivery.

- WATCH AND WAIT. **The decrease in estrogen postpartum shifts vaginal pH significantly. Many women get yeast infections after giving birth. Since you'll be in close contact with your doctor, tell her about any changes you notice, and if needed, provide a sample to be checked out at the lab.**

- STAY MOISTURIZED. **When breastfeeding, you produce more of the hormone prolactin to produce milk. High prolactin means low estrogen. Low estrogen causes vaginal dryness, which can degrade the VALT, cause microbiome dysbiosis, and lead to an infection. Dr. Horton prescribes an estrogen cream that's inserted vaginally a few times a week. It's readily absorbed into the tissue and eases dryness. Ask your doctor if this is something you can try.**

Can We Talk?

No, really, *can* we? Are we capable of talking about our vaginas without embarrassment and shame?

I certainly wasn't comfortable telling the world about mine at first. When I launched and publicized my intimate care company, I had to find the words that made it okay for me to discuss personal things in public. The more I talked about women's health care, the less shame and embarrassment I felt. Before long, I didn't hesitate to use appropriate, necessary language to empower women. At my company, we issue "public cervix announcements" to announce new products and normalize the conversation about natural body processes like discharge, odor, yeast, bacteria, and mucus. Talking the talk isn't undignified, it's liberating.

"Once, I was talking shop with a colleague at a restaurant—nothing too graphic, just using anatomical terms," said Dr. Horton. "The two women next to us were so offended by the word 'vagina' that they asked the waiter to move to another table. I felt sorry for them, because I know that women who are so afraid of saying the word are less likely to see their gynecologist if they have a problem. And if they do find the courage and make an appointment, their embarrassment makes it harder for them to explain what's wrong."

I'd love to hear women talk more about their body's natural processes, not only with their doctors, but with each other. As soon as you say, "Okay, this is embarrassing, but . . ." other women will say, "Oh, yeah, that happened to me, too." These things really aren't embarrassing, because they're normal bodily functions! Everyone feels better when things are out in the open. We are not alone in being concerned about our vaginal health and happiness. When people *don't* talk about their concerns, shame gets worse, and that takes a toll on their mental health.

Shame is another link on the GBV axis. Most of us don't speak openly about digestive issues, but if we experience them, we're preoccupied by them. Mental health issues are stigmatizing, even though they can be common. It took me a long time to admit to struggling with depression, but now I can drop, "My therapist says . . ." into the conversation without any fear of judgement. Having these troubles with your gut, brain, and/or vagina isn't a personal failing. It's not a character flaw. It just means you need to find new ways to take care of yourself.

If you're suffering but trying to give the outward appearance that you're fine and good, in the end you're just doing yourself a great disservice. Trust me on this! Silence is the opposite of self-care. When we are honest about what we're going through, we encourage others to talk about their issues. Openness relieves shame and creates a virtuous cycle of women helping women.

Next time it's on the tip of your tongue to say to a friend, "This is embarrassing, but . . ." don't hesitate. Do yourself and your friend the favor of starting what could be a life-changing conversation for you both.

HAPPY VAGINA

Keep your vagina happy and healthy with these easy solutions:

- Clean out your underwear drawer. Undergarments with fabric that nestles between the butt cheeks provide a runway for *E. coli* to get into your vagina and urethra. Bikinis and briefs *are* sexy and safe.

- Along with gut and mood probiotics, take a probiotic for women's health with multiple strains of *Lactobacilli*. This will keep your vagina slippery and leak free.

- Banish any products that use chemicals and fragrances, including bar soap. You just don't need them. Water is good enough to clean your vulva. Otherwise, look for a scent-free pH balancing wash.

- Remember: Your vagina looks and smells *fine*.

- Tone your pelvic floor by doing Kegels and core-strengthening poses the right way.

- Have an orgasm! Orgasm is a balm for your nervous, immune, and endocrine system, and masturbating as a self-love practice can also heighten desire and arousal for sex with a partner.

- Prevent UTIs by wiping front to back, peeing immediately after sex, and drinking tons of water.

- Follow the golden rule: All mammals (except for rodents) pee for the same length of time, regardless of bladder or body size. Researchers at the University of Georgia Institute of Technology discovered the "universal urination duration" for elephants, cats, deer, hippos, and humans to be 21 seconds.[10] If you take longer to pee than 21 seconds, it's a good indication that you're holding it in too long, which can increase a UTI risk. (Apologies in advance for anyone who starts obsessively counting the seconds during urination.)

TO-DO

chapter 9

LEAKS AND PATHWAYS: THE FULL DIGEST

'’ve given you a lot of information to digest so far. Like nutrients through a leaky gut with a weak GALT, you might not have absorbed all of it. That’s okay! I’m going to give you a whole-book recap about how to find whole-body harmony in this chapter.

It's a cheat sheet on the essential info about the microbiome, gut, brain, and vagina, and the pathways that keep them connected. When you get to the blissful state of homeostasis, thanks to a balanced microbiome, well-supported GBV axis, a toned vagus nerve, and a slick and thick mucus layer, you will feel light, clear, energized, and happy to be alive.

Stay that way by being an advocate for your own health. Women have no choice but to take on that responsibility, because if we don't look out for ourselves, who will? It's up to us to find receptive partners in the medical profession who will listen to us, believe us, order the tests we ask for (and the ones we don't know to ask for), and to follow up. Most importantly, we need to keep ourselves informed, by reading books like this, about how to love ourselves well.

Microbiome Essentials

- THE 100-TRILLION-CELL, four-pound microbiome of bacteria, yeast, fungi, and viruses is so diverse and so complex, it boggles the mind.

- THE LARGEST MICROBIOME in the body lives in your digestive tract, from your mouth to your anus. Smaller microbiomes live in your vagina, urinary tract, eyeballs, skin, and lungs.

- BY STRIKING A BALANCE between our good bacteria and bad bacteria, we can find homeostasis, the happy state of optimal functioning, when our gut, brain, and vagina work together to keep each other healthy and happy.

Gut Essentials

- THE GUT WALL'S INNER SKIN has three jobs: absorbing nutrients, blocking pathogens from getting into the body, and burning off pathogens.

- A HEALTHY GUT WALL'S TIGHT JUNCTIONS allow only nutrients we need for survival to pass into our bloodstream.

- A DEGRADED GUT WALL'S JUNCTIONS loosen and can let pathogens into our body. This intestinal permeability is what's known as leaky gut.

- A BALANCED GUT MICROBIOME sounds the alarm for the healthy immune system to launch an appropriate response to attack pathogens.

- AN IMBALANCED GUT MICROBIOME sounds the alarm to launch an overzealous response that attacks pathogens *and* healthy human cells.

- LEAKS can happen because of poor diet, stress, antibiotics, drinking, NSAIDs, OTC meds, recreational drugs, and caffeine, which can lead to a host of bodily malfunctions.

- GLUTEN can make your gut wall's tight junctions loosen, letting germs and toxins get into the body.

- SUPPORT GUT HEALTH by eating more plant fiber, a friendly bacteria's favorite food source.

- BENEFICIAL BACTERIA replenish themselves naturally, but take a probiotic supplement and eat fermented foods as an insurance policy to keep those populations thriving.

- THE HAPPY GUT TRIFECTA is prebiotics + probiotics = postbiotics. Eat vegetables, fruit, and grains to feed good bacteria and build up postbiotic gold nuggets.

- INTENSE EXERCISE can be counterproductive to gut health, but gentle movement helps to balance the microbiome.

- EATING ORGANIC FOODS gives the microbiome a chance to get back to normal. Perfection can be the enemy of the good, so don't go crazy. Try to avoid any food with pesticides, antibiotics, and steroids (all can be microbiome disruptors).

- AFTER A FEW WEEKS of eating organic foods and getting plenty of prebiotics and probiotics, your microbiome will be balanced and will produce lots of mucus (a good thing).

- SUPPORT GUT HAPPINESS by detoxing your life of household and cosmetic products, eating organic foods, and tamping down stress.

Brain Essentials

- THE BLOOD-BRAIN BARRIER (BBB), in a healthy system, protects the brain and blocks harmful substances from getting near it.

- MOST LIKELY, leaky brain is influenced by leaky gut's overzealous responses and rampaging cytokines that travel up the bloodstream, batter down the BBB's defenses, and get into the brain, leading to leaky brain.

- STEP ONE to a healthy brain is supporting the gut microbiome.

- EATING plant fiber (prebiotics) produces the postbiotic butyrate, an all-purpose brain booster. Every time you have an apple or an artichoke, two key prebiotics, you get a little bit smarter.

- YOUR BRAIN'S GLYMPHATIC SYSTEM only operates when you're unconscious. To power-wash the brain and take out its trash, get adequate deep sleep every night. Pro tip: For optimal brain scrubbing, sleep on your side.

- EAT ANTIOXIDANT FOODS (rainbow-colored fruits and vegetables and spices) to neutralize the free radicals that would otherwise oxidize your brain.

- STIMULATE NEW BRAIN CELL GROWTH with gentle exercise and by doing new things. The more you push your brain to expand, the healthier and happier it'll be.

- WHILE THE BRAIN DETOXES, expect some discomfort for a few days. After that, it's nothing but blue skies.

Vagina Essentials

- THE VAGINA MICROBIOME is similar to the gut's microbiome, but it's got its own blend of bacteria, dominated by *lactobacilli*.

- A HEALTHY VAGINAL PH is acidic to balance bacteria and yeasts, and ward off viruses and fungi.

- ANY SUBSTANCE that raises the vaginal pH toward alkaline could cause a bacterial imbalance.

- VAGINAL PH disrupters can include everyday items like scented, nonorganic bar soaps, cleansers, douches, lubes, condoms, and tampons.

- USE ONLY WATER to clean inside your vagina. If you want to use a cleanser on your vulva, steer toward fragrance-free, surfactant-free, paraben-free products that won't harm the *lactobacilli*.

- MAKE SURE your partner(s) clean(s) their hands and parts before they get anywhere near your vagina. Do the same with sex toys.

- WE PRODUCE half a teaspoon of discharge per day and every drop of it is precious. It rains down from the cervix and vaginal glands to slough off dead cells and keep you clean from the inside out.

- IF YOU HAVE A LEAKY VAGINA, it probably indicates an underlying condition like leaky gut that you should discuss with your doctor. Listen when your vagina tells you that something is wrong.

- TAKING A GUT PROBIOTIC SUPPLEMENT supports good bacteria everywhere. Taking a probiotic that's tailored to women's health will keep you slippery and acidic to support overall intimate health.

- KEEP YOUR VAGINA AND VULVA CLEAN during your period, a time of heightened infection risk.

- MENSTRUAL CUPS are safe and effective and better for the planet. When you clean them every twelve hours, use unscented soap and insert them with clean hands.

- TONE YOUR PELVIC FLOOR by doing Kegels and core-strengthening poses the right way.

- IMPROVE VAGINA and brain health by having an orgasm! It's a balm for your nervous, immune, and endocrine system, and it feels pretty great, too.

- THE MORE YOU TALK about your vagina, the better you'll feel and the healthier she'll be.

GBV Axis Pathways Essentials

THE NERVOUS SYSTEM

- THE FIRST BRAIN (the one in your head) is the command center for creativity, memory, and cognition; the second brain, the gut, "feels" emotion with its huge number of neurons, neurotransmitters (chemicals that allow neurons to talk to each other), and the microbiome's own nervous system.

- THE PHYSIOLOGICAL CONNECTION between the first and second brain is the "wanderer" vagus nerve (VN) that extends from the brain stem to the cervix and touches every vital organ in between. The VN is the fiberoptic cable of the body, transmitting messages to and from the brain. When the VN is strong and healthy, those lines of communication are open and the messages are clear. A weak VN sends and receives muddled messages. When messages get dropped, body functions like digestion, immunity, metabolism, and stress management break down.

- THE VN is the toggle switch between the fight-or-flight stress mode and the rest-and-digest peace mode. To turn off stress on command, practice stimulating and toning the VN with strategies like cold therapy, belly breathing, yoga, socializing, humming, laughing, and having sex.

THE IMMUNE SYSTEM

- WHEN the immune system works well, agents of infection are annihilated by antibodies and white blood cells.

- WHEN the immune system is overzealous, internal swelling can cause malfunctions throughout the body.

- MUCOSAL TISSUE, part of the lymphatic/immune system, is the slime coating on all of our inner passages, from the mouth to the vagina.

- THE GALT (the gut's own brand of mucus) and the VALT (vagina/cervix slime) provide a home for their microbiomes and a food source for good bacteria. They produce immunity cells and provide an extra layer of protection against leaks. Their slipperiness prevents bad bacteria from clumping together and sticking to the gut and vagina walls.

- THE VALT'S immune cells are so smart, they can distinguish between *not-self* pathogens they mark for death and *not-self* sperm and a growing embryo that get a hall pass and are allowed to live.

THE ENDOCRINE SYSTEM

- THE ENDOCRINE SYSTEM of glands, organs, and hormones is like a package delivery network, sending messages all over the body, along with operating instructions.

- WITH FIFTY HORMONES, all interacting with each other, the system is intertwined. One lost message can lead to total system failure.

- ENDOCRINE ORGANS: You might think the brain is the biggest and most important endocrine organ because it's chockful of glands. However, the biggest endocrine organ is the gut, and the most important one lives inside the gut—you guessed it, it's the microbiome.

- THE MICROBIOME controls how we respond to hormones, so in a way, our bacteria control how we feel (stressed, calm, happy, sad, tired, hungry, horny) and what we do (fight or flee, regulate sugar, eat, stop eating, metabolize, have sex).

- A FRIENDLY, BALANCED MICROBIOME keeps our hormones in check. We stay happy, calm, and clear. An unfriendly, unbalanced microbiome throws our hormones off-balance and could impact our overall health and feelings of wellness.

- TO REBALANCE HORMONES, increase the population of beneficial bacteria in the gut.

- SEX, with or without orgasm—even just thinking about sex, actually!—triggers a flood of serotonin, oxytocin, and dopamine, which lowers cortisol (a microbiome disruptor). Never miss an opportunity to unleash the happy hormones! Don't just do it for yourself. Do it for your bacteria, as well.

GIVE YOUR LESSER MICROBIOME SOME LOVE, TOO

I'VE FOCUSED ON THE GBV axis worlds within so far because balance in the gut, the vagina, and the urinary tract are the most impactful and important for your overall heath. If the gut microbiome is off balance, every other one will follow suit. And if you have an imbalanced vagina or bladder, you may end up feeling miserable, not just day to day, but moment to moment. I want to touch on just one more microbiome that serves and protect us—and gives us a radiant glow—namely the one that lives on your skin.

The skin is our largest organ, and it's covered, from your scalp to the toe webs, with a thousand strains of bacteria and eighty species of fungi. The specific strains are attracted to different locations—hair follicles, face, ears, chest, arm pits, elbows, back, forearms, knees, hands, feet, butt crack, groin—based on the skin's dryness, moistness, or oiliness.[1]

It might gross you out to know that there is a plush layer of fungi on your forearms and heels, and that your naval is teeming with hundreds of strains of bacteria. But I promise they have a purpose: to provide the host (you) with blanket protection. The skin microbiome keeps your epidermis at a pH of 5.0, around the same as coffee. It's not quite as acidic as the vagina, but if a pathogen lands on your face or hand, your friendly bacteria will still burn it up on contact and help heal wounds faster. The skin microbiome—in particular, the common strain *Staphylococcus epidermidis*—can block UV rays that damage your skin and cause wrinkles, although I wouldn't recommend not using sunblock.[2]

You are walking around in a head-to-toe microscopic suit of armor. To protect your coat of strains so it can help support you, do the following:

Keep a healthy gut. Scientists have linked gut balance to overall skin health.[3] By supporting your gut, you can improve the quality and glow of your skin.

Go outside. Spending time in nature and touching trees, grass, and flowers, anything green, will make your skin microbiome more diverse.[4] As you know by now, a diverse microbiome has more tools to help support healthy skin.

Clean with gentle, pH balancing products. Antimicrobial wash, basic soap, scented and chemical-laden cleansers, and hand sanitizers can potentially raise the pH of your skin and cause a dysbiosis that could negatively impact skin health and appearance.

PART 3

THE LOVE WELLNESS PLAN

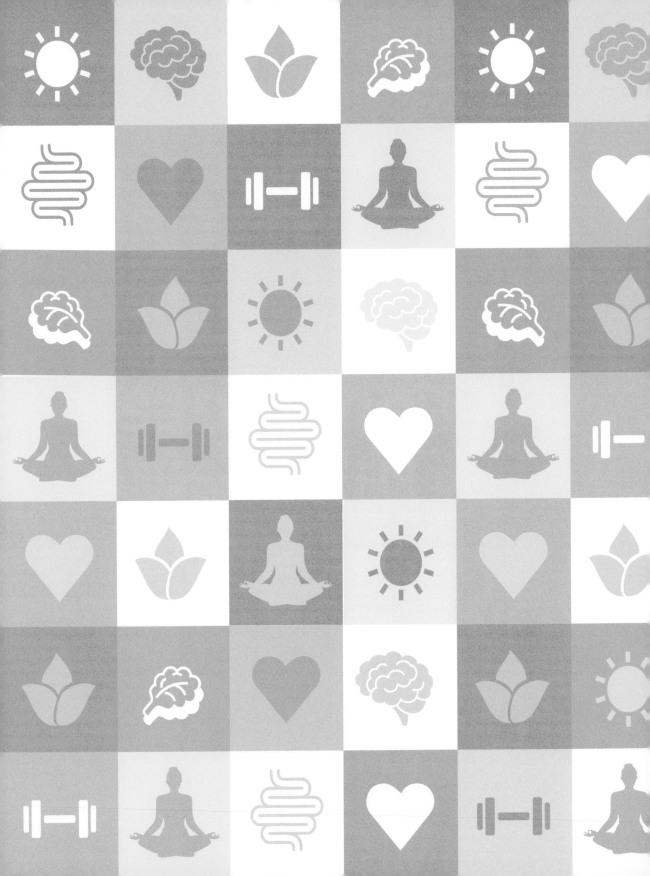

You've already learned a lot of tips—which are great when used on their own. And now, along with Certified Dietitian Nutritionist Janine Higbie, I've created a day-by-day, five-week plan, implementing all of that information and giving you the full benefits of that knowledge. Throughout the plan, you will help support the gut, brain, and vagina. By the end of it, you can reach homeostasis—whole-body balance.

In the introduction of this book, I mentioned three principles that have guided my health philosophy for the better part of a decade: (1) listen to your body, (2) it's all connected, and (3) you have to make an effort.

The Love Wellness Plan is designed so that you can hear the messages your body sends and use the GBV axis connections to your advantage. Ideally, you could keep up with it all the time. But in the real world, that's not always possible. I recommend that you do the plan every three months. The good news is that it is not hard to follow! Higbie and I agree that depravation is never the solution, so there's no calorie counting or cutting. Fewer nutrients will not get you to body harmony, but beneficial foods *will*. So you will be swapping nutrient-devoid ultraprocessed foods that wreak havoc on the gut microbiome for nutrient-dense whole foods with known benefits to our guts, brains, and vaginas. You'll start removing sabotaging toxins from your food and environment, and you'll make lifestyle tweaks and establish some new habits that seal and heal your gut, brain, and vagina in incremental, significant ways.

This is your opportunity to take control of your health and happiness from within and find harmony in the body and brain that just feels right. So let's get to it!

chapter 10

WEEK 1: PREP WEEK

Even a leak-free brain needs a minute to get used to new routines! Don't get me wrong, you *will* make changes this week that can dramatically improve your overall health by supporting your gut, brain, and vagina health, but you also need to give your brain time to adjust to the changes.

The idea beyond the seal-the-leaks plan is that the changes are so small and manageable, they won't upend your life.

Each week in the Plan includes specific actions for nutrition and lifestyle that build good habits incrementally. By accomplishing small goals, you'll get a boost of serotonin (the happy hormone) and endorphins (energy hormones) just because you're actively taking care of and loving yourself. As high serotonin means lowered cortisol, you'll instigate a healthier you just from being proud of yourself.

When to start the plan? Saturday. *This* Saturday. By launching on a weekend, you have two days to settle into it before the work week (officially) begins. Also, you'll be doing some household reorganizing, which is best done when you have some free time.

Nutrition

ACTION ITEMS ON THE LIST THIS WEEK . . .

TAPER OFF CAFFEINE

You might be having a minor heart attack right now about quitting coffee. So let me give you the good news first: You don't need to quit coffee forever. During the five weeks of the Love Wellness Plan, you're just taking a break to give your gut wall a chance to heal. Think of it as an opportunity to reduce dependency if you have one, see how you feel when you're not drinking any, and give your microbiome and vagus nerve some support.

As for why to cut back, you already know the answer to that. I have sent up warning flags about how devastating caffeine is to the microbiome and the GALT. Do you remember those old ads that said coffee was "love in every cup"? It's more like "cortisol in every cup." If you continue to drink a pot of coffee, caffeinated tea, or multiple energy drinks per day, there's no hope of plugging gut leaks. That is the cold, hard reality.

The more you rely on it, the more likely you are to experience withdrawal symptoms like headaches and fatigue. Headaches might have you reaching for NSAIDs, which are just as damaging to gut balance as caffeine. So, the goal this week is to taper off caffeine slowly to prevent the worst of withdrawal.

Higbie uses these methods to help her clients change their coffee habits:

- IF YOU DRINK CAFFEINATED BEVERAGES—coffee, tea, energy drinks—throughout the day, replace them with herbal tea or water after 1:00 p.m.

- SWITCH MORNING COFFEE OR TEA with a new blend of half-caffeinated, half-decaffeinated. On decaf coffee labels, look for the words "Swiss water process" which does not use chemicals during caffeine extraction.

- ALL COFFEE SHOULD BE ORGANIC and, if possible, third-party tested for mold, mycotoxins, and metals. Some trustworthy brands are Bulletproof, Peak Performance, Kicking Horse, and Natural Force Clean Coffee.

IT'S GOING TO HURT

EVEN A GENTLE TAPERING OFF of caffeine can cause unpleasant side effects for the first few days, so get that out of the way during prep week. In upcoming weeks, you'll be tapering down sugar and alcohol, too, which will bring more withdrawal symptoms like sleep disruptions, fatigue, brain fog, headaches, and irritability.

Stick with the plan, though. Withdrawal is a sign that your body is successfully detoxing. By the end of Week 2, the worst of it will be over. To minimize potential symptoms, stay hydrated, get plenty of rest, and go easy on yourself. This is not the time for high intensity workouts. Gentle movement is enough to get your lymph flowing and to support the detox.

As the plan unfolds, I'll have more detox recommendations that will make you feel much better right away. They counteract any pain you might have from withdrawal. It's all about balance!

START TAKING THE ESSENTIAL FIVE SUPPLEMENTS

It's hard to get the vitamins, minerals, and other nutrients you need from food alone these days because most farming practices and food processing degrade its quality; convenience eating means we're eating more preservatives and additives than ever. Nine out of ten Americans have a vitamin deficiency, and they don't even know it. If you don't feel your best, it might be a sign that you need more of the good stuff found in high quantities and top-quality vitamins and minerals. "It's great to take a 'food first' approach to get all the nutrition you need," said Higbie, "but I've yet to meet anyone who could not benefit from the Essential Five, particularly during a gut reset."

Day one (*this* Saturday), head to the store or go online and buy a month's supply of the Essential Five supplements for GBV axis health and start taking them immediately. (Of course, talk to your doctor before starting a vitamin regimen, especially if you have any health concerns. And always read the label for instructions for use and warnings.)

- A MULTIVITAMIN/MINERAL. A daily multivitamin helps fill in the dietary gaps and provides nutrients critical to a healthy immune system and mucosal tissue. Choose one that is free of dyes and additives, and make sure it includes zinc and vitamins A, C, E, and D. Take it with food in the morning because B vitamins can be energizing.

- OMEGA-3 FATTY ACIDS. Look for fish oil omega-3 supplements that have both EPA and DHA and have undergone third-party testing for mercury, environmental toxins, and contaminants. Take them with food. Vegetarians and vegans should go for algae-based omega-3 fatty acids.

- FIBER/PREBIOTICS. My favorite fiber pills, powders, and supplements are derived from psyllium husk, acacia, and vegetable fiber. You need 35 grams per day, but it's important to start slow and gradually increase your intake (otherwise you risk gastrointestinal upset). Always take fiber supplements with a *full* glass of water, or you might get constipated.

- PROBIOTICS. Ideally, you will take a gut probiotic, a mood probiotic, and a vaginal probiotic. They are designed with specific strains to support each GBV axis organ, and they're all important. I love taking probiotics with a fiber supplement because fiber is a food source for the live bacteria in a probiotic formula. The combination will support your gut with good bacteria and the food they need to thrive and produce postbiotic gold nuggets. Probiotics should be taken on an empty stomach, two hours before or after eating.

- L-GLUTAMINE. This amino acid is essential for maintaining a healthy gut lining, and it's a precursor for the body's master antioxidant, glutathione.[1] You can find L-glutamine as an ingredient in a comprehensive gut healing powder or capsule to support the intestinal tract and lining. Or you can take it as an isolated supplement, typically in powder form. Just mix it into a beverage or smoothie. Take it daily for the first four weeks of the Love Wellness Plan and discontinue once you've finished the reset. Do not take L-glutamine if you have a history of seizure disorders or liver disease.

LOCATE AN ORGANIC STORE OR FARMERS' MARKET NEAR YOU

You can't maintain a healthy gut if you're eating pesticides and additives. You can't maintain a healthy vagina if you're using intimate products with fragrance and chemical ingredients that destroy your delicate pH balance. This week, find stores near you that sell organic, chemical-free goods. You might get lucky and find one place that carries organic cosmetics, household supplies, *and* food. Organic options are more accessible than ever, even available at major supermarket chains. I happen to love going to the farmers' market on the weekends and being inspired to cook what's seasonal and what looks good. In most cities, you can get organic food from online food delivery services.

If none of those options are available to you, it's okay! Take some time this week to make your greenwash spray or soak to effectively clean all your fruits and vegetables.

SPRAY: Combine a tablespoon of lemon juice, a tablespoon of baking soda, and one cup of water in a spray bottle. Shake *gently* (it might foam). To use, spray liberally on produce, let sit for three minutes, and then rinse in cold water.

SOAK: Combine one cup of distilled white vinegar, one cup of water, and four tablespoons of salt. Place your fruits and vegetables in a bowl with the mixture and soak for ten minutes. Then rinse in cold water.

Household Clean Out

Harmful chemicals and toxins can be found in every room in your house.

Unless your couch and coffee table were made with natural, organic fibers and unfinished wood, they can release chemicals like formaldehyde (found in fabrics and building materials) and polybrominated diphenyl ethers (found in fire retardants, electronics, plastics) into the air. Even hardwood floors that have been stained or varnished can be indoor pollutants. Carpets and rugs are usually treated with fire retardants, phthalates, antistain chemicals, and pesticides. That "new carpet" and "new couch" smell is often formaldehyde.

And that's just the living room.

Don't get me started on the bedroom. If you can make one significant purchase to cut down on indoor pollutants, replace your mattress, where you spend one-third of your life, and your bedding with all-natural fabric organic versions.

Now, it would be impossible—not to mention costly—to clear your entire home of iffy items in one week or one month. And some off-gassing is low enough to be trival. So don't worry, you don't need to toss out everything in your home. I'd just recommend vacuuming carpets often, and washing drapes, throw blankets, and pillow covers with organic laundry detergent. And as you go forward in life, whenever you replace an old chair or repaint the walls, choose chemical-free items.

THIS WEEKEND, CONCENTRATE ON CLEANING OUT JUST TWO ROOMS, THE BATHROOM AND KITCHEN

IN THE BATHROOM...

- CHECK for mold in the shower and sink. If you find any, scrub it away with soap and water.

- REMOVE moldy caulk and reseal the tub. Good news: This is not nearly as hard as you might think, and the caulk guns are pretty fun!

- RUN the overhead bathroom fan often to keep the room from growing new mold. If you don't have a fan, keep a window cracked open, weather permitting.

- THROW OUT your vinyl or plastic shower curtain and liner (they often contain phthalate) and replace them with cloth curtains. Shake those out after each use!

- REPLACE drug store deodorant, shampoo, conditioner, face and body washes with natural versions, like aluminum-free deodorant instead of antiperspirant, phthalate- and paraben-free face and body wash, shampoo, and conditioner.

IN THE KITCHEN...

- REPLACE plastic storage containers and bottles for glass and steel ones. If you do keep the plastic containers, though, never use them in the microwave or freezer. Extreme temperatures can cause plastic leakage.

- INSTEAD of single-use plastic zipped baggies, use silicone reusable ones.

- SWAP aluminum foil (which can contribute to heavy metal poisoning) for parchment paper.

- REPLACE nonstick Teflon cookware with stainless steel, cast iron, or ceramic-coated pans.

- SWAP plastic cling wrap for reusable beeswax wrap.

- REPLACE cleaning products with organic products whenever possible.

What Are You Putting on Your Face?

The Environmental Working Group monitors harmful chemicals like parabens and phthalates in cosmetics at their Skin Deep website.[*] A high hazard score for a product is based on its ingredients' links to cancer, allergies, and other issues. Another resource is the Think Dirty app. Use its QR code reader to see exactly what is in the cosmetic that you are rubbing into your skin.

Toxins can accumulate over time, so start swapping out the products that you use the most. Go through your makeup bag item by item, but don't trash everything you have right away—that's just too expensive! As soon as you run out of something, switch to a cleaner product. (The one caveat is that if you're pregnant or planning to become pregnant, don't wait to replace.)

Lifestyle

MAKE SOME NEW GOOD HABITS FOR YOUR GBV AXIS

SLEEP

Start your sleep reboot with one small adjustment: Set a consistent wake time every day, including weekends. For just a month, I'm asking you not to sleep in. If you rise at the same time each morning, even on Sunday, you can avoid the dreaded Sunday Night Scaries that set you up for a bad week of sleep deprivation.

---

[*]   Go to: www.ewg.org/skindeep/

DE-STRESS

This week, get comfortable with deep breathing techniques that stem cortisol flooding and strengthen the GBV axis nervous system pathway.

Option 1: parasympathetic breathing. Inhale through the nose into the belly for a count of four, hold for a count of seven, and exhale through the mouth for a count of eight.

Option 2: box breathing. Inhale through the nose for a count of four, hold for a count of four, exhale through the mouth for a count of four, and hold for a count of four.

If you can do this for five minutes per day, great. Even one or two cycles before eating will switch on the "rest and digest" mode and will activate cellular pathways to improve digestion and absorption. Eating in "fight or flight" mode can lead to nutrient malabsorption and GI symptoms like gas and bloating.

One more de-stress goal for this week is to check out some meditation apps. You don't have to buy full access for a year now (you might want to later). Just explore a few options and try some free meditation sessions. Some recommendations are Headspace, Breathe, Calm, Happy Not Perfect, and Expectful (with a pre- and postnatal focus).

EATING WINDOW FOR PREP WEEK:

Time-restricted eating is an effective heal-and-seal tool. It's going to be helpful during prep week because it allows your body to focus on detox and resetting. It can cause lifestyle complications if you get obsessive about it. If you use it only a few days per week, you still have the flexibility for dinners or brunch out with friends and eating after a late workout.

This week, try keeping a twelve-hour eating window, followed by twelve hours of fasting.

If you're trying to conceive, are pregnant, or nursing, don't worry about fasting at all. Consult your doctor about proper nutrition.

DETOX

Establish the habit of dry brushing before each shower.

If lymphatic fluid stagnates, cellular waste and toxins just sit there. Dry brushing gets it flowing more rapidly through your body so toxins can be filtered. Side benefits are exfoliation and unclogging of pores. You can find natural bristle tools for under $5; choose one with a long handle to reach your whole back. Follow this step-by-step process:

1. Start at your feet and move up your body.

2. Move up each leg in long, light, continuing upward, sweeping movements, always toward the heart.

3. After you've brushed each leg, move on to the torso. Brushing all sides with the same continuous motion, toward the heart. If you have GI issues, brush in a clockwise motion around the lower abdomen.

4. Move on to the arms. Brush all sides, and the armpits, with the same motions, light, sweeping, and toward the heart.

5. Next, brush the neck, from the chin down, the ears down, and the back of the neck down.

6. If your skin is tingling slightly, good! If it's painful and red, you have brushed too hard.

7. Repeat once a day, before a shower (where you'll wash away the exfoliated skin cells).

SEX

HAVE AT LEAST ONE ORGASM this week for a boost of the cortisol-suppressing hormones serotonin, dopamine, and oxytocin.

If you already have a masturbation practice (and any equipment needed), hit it. Those who are vibe-curious, now is the time to go self-love shopping. Amazon has quite an inventory, as does Goop. The price range for vibrators is wide, from around $15 for the nimble bullet vibrators like the Pocket Rocket, up to around $200 for the Womanizer Duo with dual vaginal vibration and clitoral suction. What does a $200 orgasm feel like? "I can't really tell you, because I think I blacked out in the middle of it," said a friend of mine.

Be sure to use plenty of pH-balancing lube to avoid irritation and micro abrasions during masturbation and/or sex. Studies show that using lube makes it easier for women to orgasm.[2]

VAGUS NERVE STIMULATION

As a daily practice, try cold therapy. It's a proven technique to stimulate the vagus nerve and improve the all-important vagal tone and GBV axis nervous system pathways.

Dutch extreme athlete Wim Hof, aka the Iceman, has popularized an intense cold therapy regimen he claims boosts immunity and reduces inflammation. A modified version of his method that's accessible to all is comprised of the following steps:

- Take a normal shower at your preferred water temperature.

- When you've finished, turn the water as cold as it will go.

- Stand under the frigid blast for 30 seconds.

- Repeat every time you shower.

MOVEMENT

You'll probably get your twenty minutes per day of walking just from shopping and cleaning out the house of toxic products (let's not call them "goods," that just feels wrong). But throw in an additional twenty minutes per day of gentle stretching or yoga.

All week, as you get accustomed to tapering off caffeine, taking supplements, detoxing your body and home, and making lifestyle changes, check in with yourself.

How do you feel?

Have you noticed any changes?

How long did your withdrawal symptoms last?

What new practices do you like?

Which new practices do you hate and could you swap out?

Next week, you'll start eating cleaner and reducing your intake of gut disrupting foods to stop the damage.

WEEK 1 AT A GLANCE

TAPER OFF CAFFEINE
Replace with decaf after 1:00 p.m.
Morning cup should be half-caf, half-decaf
Choose organic beans
START TAKING THE ESSENTIAL FIVE SUPPLEMENTS
Multivitamin/mineral in the a.m.
Omega-3 fatty acid, taken with food
Fiber/prebiotics, taken with a full glass of water
Probiotics, taken on an empty stomach
L-glutamine, mixed into a beverage or smoothie
LOCATE STORES FOR ORGANIC FOOD AND PRODUCTS
CLEAN OUT YOUR BATHROOM AND KITCHEN OF TOXINS
In the bathroom, get rid of mold and old caulk, plastic shower curtains, and drug store brand hair and skin products. Replace with chemical and fragrance-free versions.
In the kitchen, replace plastic containers with glass and steel.
Get rid of plastic baggies and replace with silicone ones.
Buy stainless steel, cast iron, or ceramic cookware to replace Teflon.

EATING SCHEDULE

For at least a few days this week, keep eating to a 12-hour window, followed by 12 hours of fasting.

SLEEP

Set a consistent wake time every day.

DE-STRESS

Practice breathing techniques.

Choose a meditation app.

DETOX

Dry-brush before every shower.

SEX

Have at least one orgasm.

VAGUS NERVE STIMULATION

Cold therapy shower blast for 30 seconds.

MOVEMENT

20 minutes of walking per day.

20 minutes of stretching per day.

chapter 11

WEEK 2: LESS OF THE BAD STUFF

Eating foods that your body does not tolerate can lead to leaky gut just like leaky gut can bring on new food sensitivities and allergies. We should remove big offenders like gluten, alcohol, and drugs, as well as any personal triggers of inflammation and intestinal permeability to allow your body time to heal itself.

The Love Wellness Plan is not a permanent elimination diet. I don't believe it's possible to avoid whole food groups if you want to continue to live and participate in the world. After what we've all been through since the start of the pandemic, we need comfort where we can find it. And sometimes, that means having a glass of wine, a bowl of pasta, or a brownie.

To support the GBV axis body parts and find balance in the body, we need to take off the blinders. The reality is, some of the comforts we rely on are doing us, and the 100 trillion microbiotas living inside us, harm. In the long run, if poor eating and drinking cause severe symptoms and illness, we have to ask ourselves if momentary comfort is worth the damage.

If the research about certain kinds of foods/lifestyle choices were at all sketchy, I would say, "Go forth and pasta" to one and all. I wouldn't beat the organic drum so loudly. But the science is clear; the studies are conclusive. To achieve homeostasis and restore good health, we must stop consuming things that exacerbate leaks. When leaks are sealed, and the microbiome is balanced, you can reintroduce gluten, most dairy, sugar, and alcohol again, and see how that feels. After I reset my microbiome on the Plan, I made some food swaps permanent. For example, I don't eat much gluten at all anymore. I do have the occasional dessert, and I love cheese.

Nutrition

GLUTEN

Gluten, a protein found in wheat, rye, and barley, has been linked with intestinal permeability for people with celiac disease, IBS, and those who are intolerant or sensitive to it.[1] You might not be in those categories, but that doesn't mean gluten is good for your gut. It can gum up digestion for nearly everyone, causing bloating, gas, constipation, and diarrhea. Dr. Francis refers to it as an "antinutrient" because it binds to certain amino acids, vitamins, and minerals, making it harder for the body to absorb them.

Proteins called gliadins, components of gluten, have been found to release zonulin, the compound that regulates the tight junctions in the gut wall. More zonulin means increased intestinal permeability, regardless of whether you have an autoimmune condition or celiac disease.[2] A leaky gut opens the door to food intolerances, sensitivities, and allergies, as well as digestive problems and autoimmune conditions. "Symptoms of gluten sensitivity aren't limited to the gut," said Higbie. "This book delves into how gut health impacts brain and vaginal health. So it's no surprise that gluten intolerance can manifest in neurological symptoms as well. Research links gluten sensitivity to brain fog, migraines, fatigue, and even depression. Removing gluten and systematically reintroducing it is the best way to identify whether and how gluten affects you."

Cutting back on gluten is not just a matter of having only one slice of toast in the morning instead of two. It's found in foods you might expect to find it in, like barley, bulgur, bran, couscous, durum, farro, wheat germ, kamut, malt, matzah, orzo, pasta, rye, seitan, semolina, spelt, starch, tabouli, triticale, and wheat. It's also hidden in food you wouldn't expect to contain it. Hidden sources, aka "gluten you didn't see coming," are found in some candy, cheesecake, chips, prepared eggs (in restaurants), energy or granola bars, French fries, marinades, miracle burgers and meat substitutes, miso, processed lunch meats, soup/stock cubes, soy sauce, and sushi rice.

First, calculate (or approximate) how many servings of gluten you eat per day. Then try to cut that number by 75% this week.

GLUTEN SWAPS

LUCKILY, WE LIVE IN A time where restaurants and brands understand the need for gluten alternatives so there's no shortage of options.

PASTA: Try legume or chickpea pasta (higher protein and lower carb) or brown rice pasta. Once you add your favorite sauce and toppings, I swear you won't miss the gluten. Zoodles and spaghetti squash are also great options.

BREADS, TORTILLAS, CRACKERS: Try nut flour–based bread alternatives. I look for "paleo" breads in the frozen section (they work best as toast). Sourdough is a good choice, as the fermentation process breaks down almost all of the gluten. Tortillas and crackers made from nut, legume, or cassava flour are good swaps for wheat-based ones.

GRAINS: Select rice, quinoa, buckwheat, amaranth, teff, oats, sorghum, and corn instead of wheat, rye, and barley.

SOY SAUCE: Swap for coconut aminos or tamari.

SUGAR

Sugar, artificial sweeteners, and high fructose corn syrup disrupt your microbiome and contribute to systemic inflammation. These foods also change our brain chemistry. Dopamine, our "feel good" neurotransmitter, is released when we eat sugar and artificial sweeteners. When we eat them too often, the repeated exposure dampens our dopamine receptors so we need more and more sugar to get the same rush.[3] Sugar addiction is real.

Artificial sweeteners are no better for you than sugar. They're linked to gut dysbiosis and the release of endotoxins like Lipopolysaccharide (LPS) that contribute to intestinal permeability and an increased risk of inflammatory bowel disease. In lower concentrations, artificial sweeteners like aspartame and saccharin increase risk of leaky gut and at higher concentrations lead to cell death in the intestinal epithelial wall.[4]

HIDDEN SUGARS

PROCESSED AND PACKAGED FOOD LABELS are intentionally confusing, using coded language to hide sugars by using different names. Here's a decoder key for the many names for sugar:

WORDS THAT END IN "-OSE." Maltose, glucose, dextrose all mean sugar.

"SYRUP." Ingredients like brown rice syrup, malt syrup, and high fructose corn syrup are all just sugar, too.

"JUICE." It's the same thing with cane juice or fruit juice. Avoid!

HEALTHY SOUNDING "SUGAR." Beet sugar, cane sugar, coconut sugar are still sugar, even if they come from plants.

Removing sugars and artificial sweeteners, as well as other chemicals in processed foods, can reset your taste preferences and allow you to enjoy a wider range of natural flavors instead of relying on overly sweet foods. If you have a sweet tooth and find yourself craving sweets often, removing them from your diet will help reduce those cravings. Swap (in small amounts) with maple syrup, raw honey, monk fruit, stevia, or erythritol. For now, also cut back on lactose, the sugar found in dairy.

Warning: Anyone who suffers from recurring yeast infections should limit intake of even naturally occurring sugar found in fruit, honey, and maple syrup.

ALCOHOL

Here's a sobering thought: Alcohol is a neurotoxin that alters the microbiome and contributes to intestinal permeability.[5] How much do you ordinarily drink? One wine unit per day? Two? It helps to know your baseline before you mindfully decrease drinking.

Higbie recommends creating a weekly "alcohol bank." Determine the number of drinks you intend to consume while reaching your health goals. For example, if you're focusing on gut balance and optimizing fertility, keep it to under two drinks per week. (When you are restored physically and mentally by the end of the Love Wellness Plan, you can "bank" four or five drinks per week.) If you know you're only going to have two drinks per week, you can plan ahead. You might choose to save them both for a party, dinner, or event that's coming up, or for Sunday TV time. It's up to you, just don't take out more wine units than you're allotted.

BOOZE BANK

HOW MANY DRINKS ARE OKAY for your health goals this week?

Write it down: _____
(For healing and sealing, Higbie recommends two or fewer.)

Which day will you cash in your alcohol credits?

Saturday _____	Wednesday _____
Sunday _____	Thursday _____
Monday _____	Friday _____
Tuesday _____	

ULTRA-PROCESSED JUNK

Highly processed foods often contain more "food-like" ingredients than actual food. Our bodies were not designed to ingest artificial ingredients and chemicals in additives, colors, and preservatives. Fast foods have unhealthy trans fats and saturated fats that contribute to inflammation, and they're so low in fiber that they starve our good bacteria.

Any "food" that's two or more steps away from what it looked like when it came out of the ground is empty at best, damaging at worst. A potato is okay, but potato chips aren't.

MEDICINAL DISRUPTORS

Of course, if you are on prescription drugs, continue taking them. *Never go off a regimen without consulting your doctor.* However, you can probably survive without some over-the-counter convenience medicines that are known microbiome disruptors. If possible, for the next few weeks, reconsider taking these as a matter of course.

- NSAIDS. **As an alternative for pain relief, try acupressure techniques, like squeezing the web between your thumb and index finger to ease headache symptoms. Exercise is a natural analgesic, so try running up the stairs or taking a brisk walk.**

- PROTON PUMP INHIBITORS. **Acid reflux pills like Prilosec, Nexium, and Prevacid might cure heartburn, but they damage the microbiome. By taking probiotics and drinking much less coffee, you can try to control acid without drugs.**

- RECREATIONAL DRUGS. **Cannabis is legal in many states, and it has many medicinal benefits, notably as a de-stressor. However, tetrahydrocannabinol (THC), the active compound in weed, is filtered through the body's master scrub brush, the liver. Any substance that taxes our body's filtration system—especially the liver—slows down the detoxification process. Since one of the main goals of the Plan is to get the chemical sludge out, cannabis is counterproductive. You can enjoy your edibles and vape pens again *after* your gut, brain, and vagina are healed.**

TOXINS

This week, begin eating organic foods to cut out as many dietary toxins as possible.

Now that you've familiarized yourself with organic/farmers' markets near you, it's time to shift over to the holistic side. Starting *this* Saturday

(Week 2), use organic ingredients when preparing your meals to cut way back on consuming pesticides and other disrupting chemicals. Go to www.ewg.org for updates to the Clean Fifteen and Dirty Dozen lists of nonorganic produce that is particularly safe or unsafe. For proteins, look for labels that say "organic," "antibiotic-free," "grass finished" for meat, and "wild caught" for fish.

There will be times during this week, and in the upcoming weeks, when it is not possible to be sure you're eating clean food, like at a business meeting or family dinner. You don't have to be *that girl*, the one who asks the server or host about the sourcing of every ingredient. During those meals, it's fine not to worry about chemicals, and to focus on crushing the meeting or enjoying your family. The big idea here is balance, and that means not going to extremes in your thoughts or your behaviors. If you can eat organic 75% of the time, you're doing amazingly well.

NO GO, GMO: Higbie recommends to her clients to steer clear of genetically modified organisms (GMOs) because many of those crops are modified to be resistant to glyphosate, the main herbicide in Roundup, a grossly overused weed killer with toxic effects. Crops that are "Roundup ready" are heavily sprayed, which means you're getting a potentially higher toxic exposure.

Lifestyle

MAKE SOME NEW GOOD HABITS FOR YOUR GBV AXIS

SLEEP

Continue waking up at the same time each day.

NEW THIS WEEK: Set a consistent bedtime. No exceptions, even on the weekends.

Also, avoid eating within two hours of bedtime.

DE-STRESS

Continue doing five minutes per day of deep breathing using the technique of your choice.

NEW THIS WEEK: Do ten minutes per day of meditation using the app of your choice.

DETOX

Five minutes of dry-brushing before a shower.

NEW THIS WEEK: Take up to three Epsom salt or magnesium flake baths. Choose unscented salts to protect your vulvovaginal mucus layer and microbiome. Dissolve two cups of salt in a standard bathtub of water (it dissolves faster in hot water). If you have an enormous tub, use a bit more. Then soak in it for a minimum of twenty minutes.

SEX

Have two orgasms this week, alone or with a helper.

VAGUS NERVE STIMULATION

Continue cold shower therapy. If you are brave, increase the frigid blast time from thirty to forty-five seconds.

NEW THIS WEEK: Loud singing activates your vocal cords, which stimulates the vagus nerve branches on either side of your neck. If your carpool buddies object to your belting Adele from the backseat, just tell them it's your prescription medicine.

MOVEMENT

Continue walking for twenty minutes per day.

Continue doing gentle stretching or yoga for twenty minutes per day.

NEW THIS WEEK: Do three minutes of jumping to speed up the flow of lymph through your vessels. Try:

- BOUNCING ON A REBOUNDER (mini trampoline). Good for anyone who can't do hard-impact exercise, but wants to work on gentle jumping.

- STEP JUMPS. Start by standing at the foot of the stairs. Bend your knees and jump onto the bottom step. Land with both feet at once. Repeat.

- JUMPING JACKS.

- VERTICAL JUMPS.

WEEK 2 AT A GLANCE

CUT BACK ON DIETARY DISRUPTORS
Gluten: Reduce by 75%
Sugar: Reduce refined sugar by swapping with maple syrup, raw honey (and others). Cut out all artificial sweeteners.
Alcohol: Cut back to 2 drinks per week.
Ultra-processed junk: It all has to go, for now!
Swap cow cheese, yogurt, and milk with goat or sheep dairy alternatives.
Drugs: Ask your doctor about cutting back on OTC medications like NSAIDs and antacids. Stop taking recreational drugs for at least a few weeks.
Toxins: Choose organic options as much as possible.
EATING SCHEDULE
For at least a few days this week, keep eating within a 12-hour window, followed by 12 hours of fasting.
SLEEP
Set a consistent wake time.
Set a consistent bedtime.
Avoid eating within 2 hours of bedtime.

All week, as you get accustomed to reducing dietary toxins, limiting gluten, sugar, and alcohol, check in with yourself. Go to page 88 for some good questions to ask yourself.

In Week 3, the focus is on adding nutrients and delicious foods that will accelerate the health supporting process. It's all gravy from then on (well, not actual gravy).

> **EATING WINDOW WEEK 2:**
> Three or four days this week, keep a 12-hour eating window, followed by 12 hours of fasting.

DE-STRESS

5 minutes per day of deep breathing.

10 minutes per day of meditation.

DETOX

Dry-brush before every shower.

Up to 3 Epsom salt or magnesium flake baths per week.

SEX

Have at least 2 orgasms.

VAGUS NERVE STIMULATION

Cold therapy shower blast for 45 seconds.

Loud singing.

MOVEMENT

20 minutes of walking per day.

20 minutes of stretching per day.

3 minutes of jumping.

chapter 12

WEEK 3: MORE OF THE GOOD STUFF

The very good news is that the worst of the adjustment period is behind you! Over the past two weeks, you've been supporting your body by taking supplements, cutting back on disruptive foods, and removing toxins that caused leaks and imbalances.

Now, after the detox and withdrawal symptoms have ebbed, you'll have helped to seal the gut.

To review, a well-nourished gut microbiome:

- Blocks germs, toxins, and gunk from passing through the gut wall

- Maintains a healthy, slippery mucus layer

- Produces gold nugget short-chain fatty acids

- Releases neuro-transmitters to send loud and clear messages to and from the brain

- Metabolizes hormones for optimal whole-body functioning

- Tells satellite microbiomes—like the vagina's—to stay in balance

To get those benefits, eat the best stuff on Earth, that happens to come from the earth.

Nutrition

FOCUS ON PLANTS

EAT THE RAINBOW

Colorful fruits and veggies are packed with antioxidants with anti-inflammatory properties called polyphenols. Plant-based foods are categorized into six naturally occurring color groups—red, orange, yellow, green, blue/purple/black, and white/tan/brown—each with its own beneficial phytonutrients.

When you prepare a plate of food, ask yourself, "How many colors can I squeeze on here?" Diversity of color and phytonutrients is key. Higbie said, "Aim for two fistfuls of nonstarchy vegetables and fruits at two meals per day. If it's easier, just try to hit every color at least once every day." Having a vibrant salad at lunch and a steamed vegetable at dinner might be enough to get you over the rainbow. Stir fry and omelettes are other great ways to get there!

THE RAINBOW FOODS-
GBV AXIS CONNECTION

THE FOLLOWING IS A QUICK rundown of what each color does and some excellent, colorful food choices.

Red foods improve the health of your cells, GI tract, heart, hormones, and liver. Some tasty choices are apples, beans, beets, red bell peppers, blood oranges, cranberries, cherries, grapefruit (pink), goji berries, grapes, onions, plums, pomegranates, potatoes, radicchio, radishes, strawberries, raspberries, rhubarb, rooibos tea, tomatos, and watermelon.

Orange foods are full of vitamin A and improve the health of your immune system, cells, reproductive system, and skin. Great options are apricots, orange bell peppers, cantaloupe, carrots, mangos, nectarines, oranges, papayas, persimmons, pumpkin, squash, sweet potatoes, tangerines, turmeric root, and yams.

Yellow foods improve the health of your cells, brain, eyes, heart, skin, and vascular system. Eat more of these: apples, Asian pears, bananas, yellow bell peppers, corn, ginger root, lemons, millet, pineapples, star fruit, succotash, and summer squash.

Green foods improve the health of your brain, cells, skin, hormones, heart, and liver. Apples, artichokes, asparagus, avocados, bamboo shoots, bean sprouts, green bell peppers, bitter melon, bok choy, broccoli, broccolini, Brussels sprouts, cabbage, celery, cucumbers, edamame, green beans, green peas, green tea, all leafy greens, limes, okra, green olives, pears, snow peas, watercress, and zucchini.

Blue/purple/black foods improve the health of your cells, brain, heart, and liver. Go for these choices: purple bell peppers, berries, red cabbage, purple carrots, cauliflower, eggplant, figs, grapes, olives, plums, potatoes, prunes, raisins, and forbidden (black) rice.

Finally, white/tan/brown foods are anticancer, antimicrobial, and help out your cells, GI tract, heart, hormones, and liver. Have more of these: apples, cauliflower, cocoa, coconut, dates, garlic, jicama, legumes, mushrooms, nuts, onions, pears, sauerkraut, seeds, shallots, soy, tahini, tea, and whole grains.

In addition to focusing on increasing rainbow fruits and vegetables, legumes are an excellent source of plant-based protein, vitamins, and minerals—and fiber. Lentils, beans, and peas are so packed with dietary fiber, a serving or two per day will help you hit your daily fiber goal of 35 grams. It's best to gradually increase legume intake, though, to give your body a chance to adjust. If you add too much fiber too fast, it could lead to constipation, painful gas, and bloating, especially if you don't drink enough water. We want the toxins out, not stuck in your gut. Many toxins find their way out in urine, so keep your internal streams flowing by drinking plenty of filtered water and herbal tea. A guideline for how much to drink is: half your body weight in pounds = your daily fluid ounce goal. If you weigh 140 pounds, try to drink 70 fluid ounces per day.

QUALITY CARBS

Refined and processed carbohydrates (flours, breads, pastas) deserve their bad reputation. But don't paint all carbs with the same brush. We need *quality* carbs to energize our cells and feed our microbiome.

Foods that we humans might think of as humble—potatoes, bananas, rice, white beans, oats, peas, and lentils—are like a luxury banquet for our good bacteria. These "resistant starches" pass through the small intestines without being digested (hence, "resistant"). When they reach the large intestines, they ferment into prebiotics that feed good bacteria. (Resistant starches have other benefits, too, like helping to improve insulin sensitivity and overall blood sugar balance.)

For some foods like rice and potatoes, cooling them after cooking helps to increase resistant starch, and reheating won't undo those benefits. Other foods have higher resistant starch in their raw form like oats, unripe bananas, and some legumes. This is why overnight oats (uncooked) are higher in resistant starch than cooked oatmeal.

BEAN BATH

SOAKING AND SPROUTING LEGUMES, NUTS, and seeds removes certain antinutrients like phytate, goitrogens, lectins, and thiaminases that block the absorption of beneficial nutrients. Soaking beans has its own particular benefit to make them more tolerable (i.e., less gassy).

To boost the nutrient power of most legumes, nuts, and seeds:

Measure out how much you'll need and place them into a bowl.

Cover the food with at least an inch of water.

Soak them for at least seven hours or, preferably, overnight.

Drain and cook them within the next one or two days (they do not last as long once soaked).

GUT SUPERFOODS

Glutamine, one of the Essential Five daily supplements that you've been taking for the past two weeks, helps to produce glutathione, your body's "master antioxidant."

But there are plenty of superfoods you can add to your diet to help out.

An excellent source of collagen, trace minerals, *and* important amino acids like glutamine, glycine, and proline is bone broth. Next time you make a soup like the ones in the next section of this book, use high quality organic, grass-fed bone broth instead of boxed stock. Source and quality matter when it comes to buying any animal product. When nonorganic bones are cooked, toxins and heavy metals (like lead) leach into the broth.

In another category of superfood, fermented plant foods, like kimchi, pickles, and sauerkraut, and fermented soybeans like natto, tempeh, and miso, contain live beneficial bacteria that can populate your gut and improve your microbiome and overall health. If your body can tolerate dairy, add fermented products like yogurt and kefir into your diet, but steer clear of nonfermented dairy like milk, cream, ice cream, and cheese. Sheep and goat yogurts are potentially less inflammatory and better tolerated than cow dairy. Coconut yogurt and kefir are great nondairy alternatives that still provide beneficial probiotics.

Sadly, fermented wine and beer do not contain probiotics.

Lifestyle

MAKE SOME NEW GOOD HABITS FOR YOUR GBV AXIS

SLEEP

Wake up at the same time each day.

Go to bed at the same time each day.

Avoid eating within two hours of bedtime.

NEW THIS WEEK: Shut off all electronic devices an hour before bedtime. Dr. Breus calls this "the power-down hour." The blue light from phones, tablets, and computers suppresses melatonin (the sleep hormone) secretion, so turning off devices gives your endocrine system a chance to do its job, undisrupted by technology.

DE-STRESS

Five minutes per day of deep breathing using the technique of your choice.

Ten minutes per day of meditation using the app of your choice.

NEW THIS WEEK: Ten minutes per day of nature exposure. Just a few minutes of being in nature, among trees and birds, dramatically lowers cortisol levels. It works for urban dwellers (like me), too. Any patch of green will do its magic on your nervous system. And there's a bonus: If you can take off your socks and shoes and walk barefoot on grass, the calming effects are multiplied.

DETOX

Five minutes of dry-brushing before a shower.

Three weekly Epsom salt baths, using two cups of salt in the water.

NEW THIS WEEK: Sweat. Either take a gentle hot yoga class, spend ten minutes in a sauna, or use an infrared blanket. Only one sweat session per week is enough. Too much and you could get dehydrated, which prevents detox from happening. Regardless of your chosen sweat method, always drink sixteen ounces of filtered water afterward.

Infrared blankets are like having a personal sauna in a sleeping bag. Velcro yourself into it, turn it on, and the electromagnetic radiant light, invisible to the human eye, heats you up from the inside, making you sweat. I use my infrared blanket without fail once a week for half an hour, and I always feel better afterwards. They are available at online retailers at various price points—starting at $150 and going into the thousands. If I paid for a three-month package of infrared sauna sessions at a spa, it would cost the same as a mid-range blanket. So buying one pays for itself—if you use it. If it just gathers dust in a closet, it's not.

SEX

Have three orgasms this week, alone or with a helper.

VAGUS NERVE STIMULATION

Cold shower therapy. If you are truly dedicated, extend your frigid blast from forty-five to sixty seconds.

Sing loud, sing proud. Belt out a few songs per day while getting dressed.

NEW THIS WEEK: Massage. You don't have to go to a spa and pay a hefty price (although if that is in your budget, go for it). Massage can stimulate the vagus nerve and perk up the lymphatic system to aid in detox. Just stroke your neck from the notch behind your ears in a downward motion toward the collarbone twenty times. Combine it with OM chanting for twice the toning.

MOVEMENT

Walking for twenty minutes per day.

Gentle stretching or yoga for twenty minutes per day.

Three minutes of jumping on a rebounder, jumping jacks, or vertical jumps. Hold your boobs if necessary.

NEW THIS WEEK: More of the same. If your energy levels are good, increase the length of time you spend walking, stretching, and jumping.

WEEK 3 AT A GLANCE

FOCUS ON PLANTS

Eat the rainbow. Try to hit every color at least once a day.

Gradually increase fiber from vegetables and fruits to get to 35 g per day (and remember to hydrate throughout!).

Choose quality carbs, especially resistant starches like potatoes, rice, and oats.

Experiment with gut superfoods like organic bone broth and fermented plants and legumes, sheep and goat yogurts, and fermented coconut products.

EATING SCHEDULE

For at least a few days this week, keep eating to a 10-hour eating window, followed by 14 hours of fasting.

SLEEP

Set a consistent wake time.

Set a consistent bedtime.

Avoid eating within 2 hours of bedtime.

Shut off all devices an hour before bed.

DE-STRESS

5 minutes per day of deep breathing.

After a solid week of adding color to your diet, drinking lots of water, and increasing your fiber, you are now a champion pooper, and are well on your way to qualifying for the side hustle of stool donation. As always, check in with yourself by running through the questions on page 74.

Next week, you'll focus on adjusting to healthy fats and quality proteins, the final nutritional action items to get your body in balance.

EATING WINDOW WEEK 3:
Three or four days this week, keep a 10-hour eating window, followed by 14 hours of fasting.

10 minutes per day of meditation.
10 minutes per day of nature exposure.
DETOX
Dry-brush before every shower.
Up to 3 Epsom salt or magnesium flake baths per week.
Sweat gently once a week.
SEX
Have at least 3 orgasms.
VAGUS NERVE STIMULATION
Cold therapy shower blast for 60 seconds.
Loud singing.
Neck massage.
MOVEMENT
20 minutes of walking per day.
20 minutes of stretching per day.
3 minutes of jumping.

chapter 13

WEEK 4: BLISS IS YOURS

By the end of Week 4, if you are taking the Essential Five supplements, limiting your alcohol, caffeine, gluten, sugar, and nonorganic foods intake, eating more colorful plants, fiber-rich legumes and resistant starches, and hitting all of your lifestyle goals, your body is primed for optimal functioning: Homeostasis is in sight!

During the earlier weeks of the Love Wellness Plan, the focus was on one of the three macronutrients: carbohydrates. This week, the focus shifts to the other two: fats and protein. Certain fats can work their magic on your gut and brain to support a healthier you. Lean proteins are necessary to keep the gut wall sealed, to aid in detox, and provide the energy you need now that you're feeling healthier.

Just one final push to go, and you have a body in balance. Some of the significant things you're doing by following the Plan support your digestive, mental, and vaginal health, which means:

Less bloating, gas, and constipation.

Lowered risk of brain fog, anxiety, and depression.

Lowered risk of vaginal and urinary tract infections.

There's one way to go from here: forward in life, happiness, and health.

Nutrition

FOCUS ON FATS AND PROTEIN

ANTI-INFLAMMATORY FATS

For three weeks now, you've been supplementing with omega-3 fatty acids. Keep it up. Taking fish oil or algae capsules goes part of the way to balancing a healthy ratio of omega-3s with their cousin omega-6 fatty acids. Evidence suggests that humans evolved to eat an omega-6 to omega-3 ratio of about 1:1. Western diets today have an imbalanced ratio of 16:1, with omega-6s far outpacing omega-3s.[1]

Where do all those omega-6s come from? These fatty acids are found in ubiquitous industrial seed oils—"vegetable oils" like corn, canola/rapeseed, soybean, and safflower—in nearly every processed and packaged food, even in popular oat milk (go for almond milk instead). Check the labels. They sound friendly but they are among the worst offenders out there.

That doesn't mean omega-6s are bad. It is essential that humans get adequate supplies of both omega-3s and omega-6s, since they play an important role in regulating our immune system and healing from injury. But too much omega-6 may contribute to an overzealous immune response, which can impair our overall health and upset the delicate balance of our microbiome.

It's important to both increase your intake of omega-3s *and* greatly reduce your intake of omega-6s. Taking fish oil alone isn't enough. The two omega types compete for the same pathways and enzymes, so unless you decrease omega-6s, you're not going to get the full benefits of adding omega-3s, through food or supplements.

What's more, one source of omega-3 is preferable to others. Although it's beneficial to eat plant-based sources like flax seeds and walnuts, they're not enough either. They don't convert well to brain-essential DHA and EPA. Fish, fish oil, or cod liver oil feed the brain the fatty acids it craves. (Vegans and vegetarians can take an algae-based omega-3 oil.) To remember optimal low mercury sources, use the acronym SMASH: salmon, mackerel, anchovies, sardines, herring. Avoid larger fish like shark, swordfish, marlin, tilefish, bigeye tuna, king mackerel, orange roughy. Big fish eat little fish. The higher up the food chain fish get, the more bioaccumulation and biomagnification of mercury they can have.

Other healthy fats are monounsaturated and can be found in olives, olive oil, avocados, nuts, and seeds. Unrefined oils (meaning, the oil goes straight from the press into the bottle) like extra virgin olive oil are great for dressings, drizzling over already cooked food, or dipping. But because of their low smoke point, they become damaged and lose their nutritional value at high temperatures. Don't keep oils above or near the stove, oven, or other heat sources for that reason. For cooking at high temperatures, use avocado oil, coconut oil, or ghee, instead of olive oil.

HERBS FULLY LOADED

HERBS AND SPICES ADD MORE than just flavor to food. They are full of antioxidants and immune-supporting substances. Using a wide variety of spices and herbs can keep healthy eating interesting. A new spice profile can make a familiar dish new again. Use them liberally.

Immune support: turmeric, cayenne pepper, chili powder, cilantro, ginger, nutmeg, and paprika

Digestive aids: cinnamon, cumin, and dill

Antioxidants: cloves, oregano, rosemary, and thyme

POWER PROTEINS

Amino acids, the building blocks of protein, play a critical role in liver detox and the synthesis of neurotransmitters. They maintain the integrity of the epithelial tissue that lines the digestive tract and help support gut health. Protein is important at every meal for turning off ghrelin (the hunger hormone) and promoting prolonged satiety.[2]

The rare woman gets as much protein as she needs. For a long time, the U.S. recommended daily allowance (RDA) of protein has been calculated using this formula: 0.8 grams of protein per kilograms of body weight per day. However, the RDA does not reflect ideal or optimal levels. Fortunately, we have a large body of current research that confirms a healthier formula for a sedentary healthy weight person: 1.2 to 1.8 grams per kilogram of body weight per day. A 140-pound woman weighs 63.5 kilograms. Her protein need is 63.5 x 1.2 or 76.2 grams. If she's more active, 63.5 x 1.8 or 114.3 grams per day. Higbie recommends splitting up daily protein by having 20 to 30 grams per meal and throwing in a 10- to 15-gram snack.

The optimal protein RDA is higher for women who are very active, athletic, overweight, trying to lose weight or gain muscle, or are pregnant or lactating.

Not just any protein will do. Choose lean, clean sources like wild caught fish, organic eggs, and plant-based protein like organic tofu or tempeh, lentils, chickpeas, beans, quinoa, nuts, and seeds. Quality animal protein in moderation is absolutely part of a healthy diet. Higbie reports that, in her practice, she often sees people relying too heavily on animal protein and not getting enough plant-based sources that contain fiber and phytonutrients. Animal flesh doesn't offer much nutritionally besides protein and fat. Toxins and pesticides are fat-soluble so they can be stored in the fatty tissues of animals (and humans). Choose lean meats, especially if you're not able to control the quality (grass-fed/finished, pasture-raised).

Founding father Thomas Jefferson once wrote, "I have lived temperately, eating little animal food, and that, not as an aliment so much as a condiment for the vegetables, which constitute my principal diet." Centuries later, author Mark Hyman, MD, repurposed Jefferson's words and came up with the phrase "condi-meat" as a way to remind people that meat should not take up more space on the plate than a condiment in an otherwise plant-based meal.

Lifestyle

MAKE SOME NEW GOOD HABITS FOR YOUR GBV AXIS

SLEEP

Wake up at the same time each day.
Go to bed at the same time each day.

Avoid eating within two hours of bedtime.

Shut off all devices an hour before bedtime.

NEW THIS WEEK: Get fifteen minutes of sunlight exposure first thing in the morning. Early morning sun signals to the brain that a new day has come. Have your half-caf coffee or tea outside or take a quick walk before breakfast.

DE-STRESS

Five minutes per day of deep breathing using the technique of your choice.

Ten minutes per day of meditation using the app of your choice.

Ten minutes per day of nature exposure.

DETOX

Five minutes of dry-brushing before a shower.

Three weekly Epsom salt baths, using two cups of salt.

Once a week sweating, in a sauna, with an infrared blanket, or at a gentle hot yoga class.

SEX

Have three orgasms this week, alone or with a helper.

Combine sex with loud moaning. Sexy yummy vibrating sounds are just as good as humming, OM chanting, and singing to stimulate the vagus nerve and switch to parasympathetic mode. When in that state, your reproductive organs are relaxed, allowing increased blood flow, which is the definition of sexual arousal.

"I tried this trick when masturbating, because I didn't want to frighten my boyfriend," said a friend of mine. "I made throaty, guttural noises, increasing volume the closer I got to coming. I swear that my orgasm was twice as intense because of it. I think it's because the noises vibrated my vagus nerve at the same time as my vibrator stimulated the pudendal nerve in my clitoris." Try as I might, I could not find a scientific study to confirm that orgasms are stronger when making loud noises, but it's important research we can all do in the privacy of our own homes. (Report back. I'm collecting anecdotal data.)

> EATING WINDOW
> WEEK 4:
> Three or four days this week, keep an 8-to-10 hour eating window, followed by 14-to-16 hours of fasting.

VAGUS NERVE STIMULATION

Cold shower therapy. If you are truly dedicated, extend your frigid blast to sixty seconds.

Sing loud, sing proud. Belt out a few songs per day while getting dressed.

Neck massage. Twenty strokes while OM chanting.

NEW THIS WEEK: Social connection and laughter. The parasympathetic nervous system is called "safe and social" mode. When we connect with loved ones, we create an upward spiral of positive emotion and increased vagal tone. Because people have different comfort levels at this point in the pandemic, this can look different! Whether it's a Zoom hangout or an IRL dinner depleting your alcohol bank, there are plenty of ways to spend quality time with loved ones.

MOVEMENT

Walking for at least twenty minutes per day.

Gentle stretching or yoga for at least twenty minutes per day.

Two sessions of three minutes each of jumping on a rebounder, jumping jacks, or vertical jumps. Invest in a good sports bra or hold your boobs if necessary.

Now that you are cooking with monosaturated oil, overseeing intake of omega-6s, and steering away from steer (meaning cow flesh) to eat more plant proteins, your nutritional reset is complete. After four weeks of supplementing, healthy eating, and lifestyle goals that have drastically cut down on stress, eliminated toxins, and enabled you to clean out your brain every night, you are no doubt feeling as balanced as ever.

Congrats! You have done it. Homeostasis is yours. The gut, brain, and vagina are balanced.

Now that you've reset and are in balance, you have a clean slate. What do you want to draw on it? Do you want to go back to the way things were or proceed on the balanced path? There is a healthy middle ground, what I call Ongoing Balance, coming up in the next chapter.

WEEK 4 AT A GLANCE

FOCUS ON HELPFUL FATS

Increase omega-3 fatty acids.

Reduce omega-6 fatty acids.

EXPERIMENT WITH HERBS AND SPICES

POWER UP WITH PROTEIN

Calculate your protein need and distribute grams over 3 meals per day.

Decrease animal proteins.

Increase plant proteins.

EATING SCHEDULE

For at least a few days this week, keep an 8- to 10-hour eating window, followed by 14 to 16 hours of fasting.

SLEEP

Set a consistent wake time.

Set a consistent bedtime.

Avoid eating within 2 hours of bedtime.

Shut off all devices an hour before bed.

10 minutes of morning sun exposure.

DE-STRESS

5 minutes per day of deep breathing.

10 minutes per day of meditation.

10 minutes per day of nature exposure.

DETOX

Dry-brush before every shower.

Up to 3 Epsom salt or magnesium flake baths per week.

Sweat gently once a week.

SEX

Have at least 3 orgasms.

If inspired, turn up the volume.

VAGUS NERVE STIMULATION

Cold therapy shower blast for 60 seconds.

Loud singing.

Neck massage.

Socializing and laughing.

MOVEMENT

20 minutes of walking per day.

20 minutes of stretching per day.

2 sessions of 3 minutes of jumping.

chapter 14

WEEK 5: ONGOING BODY BLISS

believe in the 21/90 rule, meaning that it takes 21 days to make a habit and 90 days to cement it in. After 28 days on the Love Wellness Plan, you are well on your way. Your microbiomes are balanced and supporting your gut, brain, and vagina health.

I hope some of the lifestyle goals like meditation, detoxing, and good sleep hygiene are locked in or on their way to being automatic.

Hitting reset doesn't mean that you will stay sealed forever. Leaks can spring anew, especially if you revert to the old ways of being, eating, drinking, sleeping, as before. Our health is always on a tight rope, always one misstep away from imbalance. That said, if we're too obsessed with the care and feeding of our microbiome, we can become needlessly stressed out. If we're too fixated on eating a rainbow of plants, we'll miss out on the joy of a rare (meaning temperature and frequency) juicy cheeseburger.

Balance is bigger than what's happening inside our gut. It's our entire life.

Loving yourself well also means giving yourself permission to find a middle ground that preserves GBV axis harmony and allows for occasional indulgences. If you're eating well and taking supplements, it's okay to have a couple of gin and tonics on Saturday night.

The ultimate goal for ongoing balance is to have it all: good health and fun. Part of the Plan is doing a weekly check in about how you feel. If you keep up that one practice and ask yourself what's working for you and what isn't, you'll know (not feel or guess) how to tip yourself back into balance if you get wobbly.

Nutrition

KEEP IT UP

If you don't miss caffeine and alcohol and feel good without them, maybe don't dive into a pot of coffee or a bottle of wine just yet. See how life is without them for a while. Excess sugar is never good for you. But I get it: freshly baked cookies make life worth living. Play with moderation and see how you feel. And then follow whichever path makes you feel sparkly.

Foods and food chemicals that you *know* trigger an overzealous immune response and could lead to leaky gut, brain, and vagina, should not be part of your daily diet—because they make you feel like poop (and not the quadruple S kind). Depending on the status of your overall health, your goals, and your reactions to foods, you should consider completely cutting out food triggers or have them no more than a few times per week. You can stay true to the principles of a balanced life by allowing for some flexibility about self-imposed rules. Otherwise, you'll over-"rule" yourself out of opportunities to connect with other people. Be real with yourself, and if you notice symptoms again, if your health goals are slipping, it's time to rein it in.

EATING OUT

If the majority of your meals helps you feel your best, you'll be in good shape. If there's something on the menu you love but maybe isn't beneficial for your gut, brain, and vagina, try to share it with someone else at the table. Or ask that it be brought out at the same time as your healthy main course. Eat the healthy food first, and then go for the French fries once you're already almost full.

When eating family style, fill your whole plate before you start eating anything—as opposed to sampling many dishes without any sense of portion control—and then start with the plants. This strategy helps with overall weight management, but it's also great for keeping track of the foods that you love in the moment but pay for later.

When you're not in full control of what you eat, like at a dinner party, choose the leanest cuts of meat. Toxins and pesticides are concentrated in fat. Reducing animal fat can reduce potential exposure. Lastly, if the meal is outside your eating window, don't stress out about it. Don't let perfection—in food choice or timing—be the enemy of the good.

TO PORTION YOUR PLATE . . .

- Half should be non-starchy vegetables.

- One fourth should be starchy vegetables, fruit, legumes, or whole grains.

- One-fourth should be protein and fats.

REINTRODUCTION

Humans do well on a varied healthy diet, both from a nutrient perspective and by reducing the risk of creating food triggers. You're less likely to get bored with your new way of eating if you're constantly mixing it up. So, in the spirit of variety, now is the time to reintroduce foods that you removed from your diet in the Plan, like cow cheese, pasta, and alcohol, for example. With a clean slate, you're in a great position to test your body's ability to tolerate these foods.

Conduct a science experiment on yourself by reintroducing one food group at a time and tracking how you feel. Eat two or three servings in one day and wait forty-eight hours. Then run through an assessment of how you feel. Use the following chart as a guide.

If you have a reaction to a reintroduced food, Higbie recommends going off it for six months before trying it again. If you don't have a re-

	DAY 1	DAY 2	DAY 3	DAY 4
Time				
Food				
Joint/Muscle Aches				
Headaches/Pressure				
Nasal or Chest Congestion				
Kidney/Bladder Function				
Skin				
Energy Level				
Sleep				
Other Symptoms				

LOVE YOURSELF WELL

action, enjoy it in moderation. The "all clear" is not carte blanche to eat or drink the particular food or beverage with the same frequency that got you into a pre–Love Wellness Plan mess. When we eat the same things over and over, the body can become sensitized to that food or to a certain component of that food, and we can re-create an allergy, intolerance, or sensitivity.

Don't re-dig the same hole and fall back into it. The balanced life is about self-knowledge, not self-sabotage.

THE ESSENTIAL FOUR

Continue taking a multivitamin/mineral, omega-3 fatty acid supplements, probiotic supplements, and daily fiber gummies, pills, or powder.

Now that you've taken your life back into your own hands, you can discontinue the l-glutamine supplement. If you want to replace it with something, take additional vitamin D3 to supplement what's in your multivitamin/mineral. First, though, ask your doctor to run a simple blood test called "25,OH-D" to determine your vitamin D level and whether supplementation is needed. Optimal levels are between 40–80 nmol/L. It's generally safe to start with a total of 2000 IU of total supplemental vitamin D3 (cholecalciferol) daily, but consult your doctor to determine what's best for you.

FOR THOSE WHO LIKE STRUCTURE . . .

Here are some general guidelines for your ongoing balanced nutrition:

- 25 to 35 grams of fiber per day

- Fermented foods daily

- 20 to 30 grams of protein per meal

- 12 ounces per week of low-mercury fatty fish

- Only plant sources for fats, like avocado, nuts, seeds, olives, and coconut

- Minimal intake of inflammatory seed oil. Check the labels of all packaged foods, dressings, marinades, and prepared foods for hidden vegetable oils.

Lifestyle

SLEEP

Wake up at the same time each day.

Go to bed at the same time each day.

Avoid eating within two hours of bedtime.

Shut off all devices an hour before bedtime.

Get fifteen minutes of sunlight exposure first thing in the morning.

Try adding melatonin supplements to help with occasional sleeplessness.

DE-STRESS

Five minutes per day of deep breathing using the technique of your choice.

Up to fifteen minutes per day of meditation using the app of your choice. At this point, you'd feel weird if you didn't do fifteen minutes per day. Make it permanent.

Ten minutes per day of nature exposure.

DETOX

Five minutes of dry brushing before a shower.

Three weekly Epsom salt baths, using two cups of salt.

Once a week sweating, in a sauna, with an infrared blanket, or at a gentle hot yoga class.

SEX

Have three orgasms this week, alone or with a helper. And get loud about it!

VAGUS NERVE STIMULATION

Cold shower therapy. If you are truly dedicated, extend your frigid blast to sixty seconds.

Sing loud, sing proud. Belt out a few songs per day while getting dressed.

Neck massage. Twenty strokes while OM chanting.

Keep seeing loved ones and laughing, as often as possible. What's the point of healing and sealing if you don't enjoy your health and happiness, and share the love with others?

MOVEMENT

Walking for at least twenty minutes per day.

Gentle stretching or yoga for at least twenty minutes per day.

Two sessions of three minutes of jumping on a rebounder, jumping jacks, or vertical jumps. Hold your boobs if necessary.

NEW AND ONGOING: Exercise. Cortisol stress isn't as big a danger with a balanced microbiome and robust mucus layer that you have now re-stored on the Plan. So you can resume more strenuous exercise for up to an hour per session, three times per week. More than that, and you can compromise your microbi-ome and gut wall again. Do what works best for you.

The Love Wellness Plan gave you the foundation for a new life in balance. Whatever you do next will build upon that foundation. As always, check in with yourself every week, now and going forward, about how you feel, what feels good and bad, and what you can do to feel even more blissful?

You know what—and "why exactly"—to do now.

It's up to you to be your own best advocate for your health and happiness.

No one else can or should love you as well as you love yourself.

> **EATING WINDOW ONGOING:**
> Try circadian rhythm time-restricted eating or not eating after the sun goes down. Depending on the season, you'll have a longer or shorter eating window.
>
> If you feel good about the way you've been eating thus far, stick with it. Several times a week, restrict eating to 8-to-10-hour windows, followed by 14 to 16 hours of fasting.

WEEK 5 AT A GLANCE

STRIKE A BALANCE BETWEEN GOOD HEALTH AND GOOD TIMES

Reintroduce limited caffeine, but only if you miss it.

Increase alcohol units to 4 per week.

Have the occasional cookie.

EAT OUT

Steer toward plants, no matter where you are.

Mind your portions.

FOOD TRIGGER WARNINGS

Slowly reintroduce gluten, cow dairy, and sugar.

To assess for intolerance and sensitivities, use the tracker above.

SUPPLEMENT UPDATE

Stop taking l-glutamine.

Keep taking everything else that is working for you.

EATING SCHEDULE

Circadian rhythm time-restricted eating. Don't eat when the sun goes down.

For at least a few days this week, keep an 8-to-10-hour eating window, followed by 14 to 16 hours of fasting.

SLEEP

Set a consistent wake time.

Set a consistent bedtime.

Avoid eating within 2 hours of bedtime.

Shut off all devices an hour before bed.

15 minutes of morning sun exposure.

Melatonin supplements, as needed.

DE-STRESS

5 minutes per day of deep breathing.

15 minutes per day of meditation.

10 minutes per day of nature exposure.

DETOX

Dry-brush before every shower.

Up to 3 Epsom salt or magnesium flake baths per week.

Sweat gently once a week.

SEX

Have at least 3 orgasms.

Turn up the volume with your moaning.

VAGUS NERVE STIMULATION

Cold therapy shower blast for 60 seconds.

Loud singing.

Neck massage.

Socializing and laughing.

MOVEMENT

20 minutes of walking per day.

20 minutes of stretching per day.

2 sessions of 3 minutes of jumping.

Exercise up to 3 times a week.

JANINE HIGBIE ON NUTRITION FOR HOPEFUL, EXPECTANT, AND NEW MOMS

My specialty is working on the nutrition of women who are planning to get pregnant (including egg freezing and artificial reproductive technologies), are currently pregnant, and are recovering from it. The Love Wellness Plan is perfectly healthy for women at every stage of reproduction.

IF YOU'RE TRYING TO CONCEIVE, your diet and lifestyle choices in the four months leading up to conception influence egg quality, fertility, and miscarriage risk. If you are planning for pregnancy or prepping for artificial reproductive technology, much is out of your control, but diet is one factor you can take charge of. Talk to your doctor: Absolute essentials are prenatal multivitamins, DHA/EPA, and probiotics. Every nutrition recommendation in the Plan is good for you, including gentle time-restricted eating. I'd even say that microbiome balance is essential. The vaginal microbiome impacts hormone production within the ovaries and their overall health. To increase your odds of conception, take a vagina specific probiotic and eat lots of plant fiber to feed your good bacteria.

IF YOU'RE PREGNANT, do not limit your eating window during pregnancy. Listen to your body and eat when you're hungry! I don't mean to be scary, but the fact is, your diet during pregnancy can impact your child's future risk for long-term chronic disease. As many nutrient requirements increase significantly during pregnancy, you really don't have room in your diet for empty calories. Following the advice in the plan—focusing on fiber-rich, gut-supportive plants, anti-inflammatory fats, and lots of protein—will help support your baby's growth and development. Protein intake needs to be increased during this time to a minimum of 80 grams per day in the first half of pregnancy, and 100 grams per day in the second half of pregnancy. Don't freak out if you're not eating your best during the first trimester when food aversions peak and you seemingly can tolerate only carbs. This happens often! The good news—your baby will pull on your nutrient stores if your diet isn't providing sufficient nutrition. If you've done the work prior to conception, you'll be in great shape.

IF YOU'RE NURSING, know that significant and increased calorie demands extend into the postpartum time, particularly if you're nursing. For example, healthy weight women need an additional 300 calories per day during pregnancy and an additional 500 calories while nursing compared to prepregnancy intake. Just like in pregnancy, the foods you eat while nursing nourish both you and your baby. You should always consult your health care practitioner before starting new supplements while pregnant or nursing, but I always recommend continuing prenatal supplements for at least six months postpartum or throughout nursing, whichever is longer. Some nursing nutrient demands—like vitamins A, B2, B6, B12, C, selenium, zinc—increase compared to pregnancy, so those supplements are an important safety net. The quality of your diet can also impact the nutrient content of your breast milk. This is not a time for cutting foods or calories. This is a time to focus on a varied nutrient-dense diet like the Love Wellness Plan.

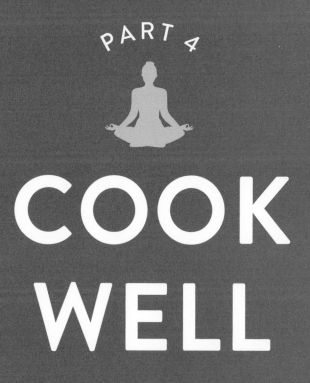

COOK
WELL

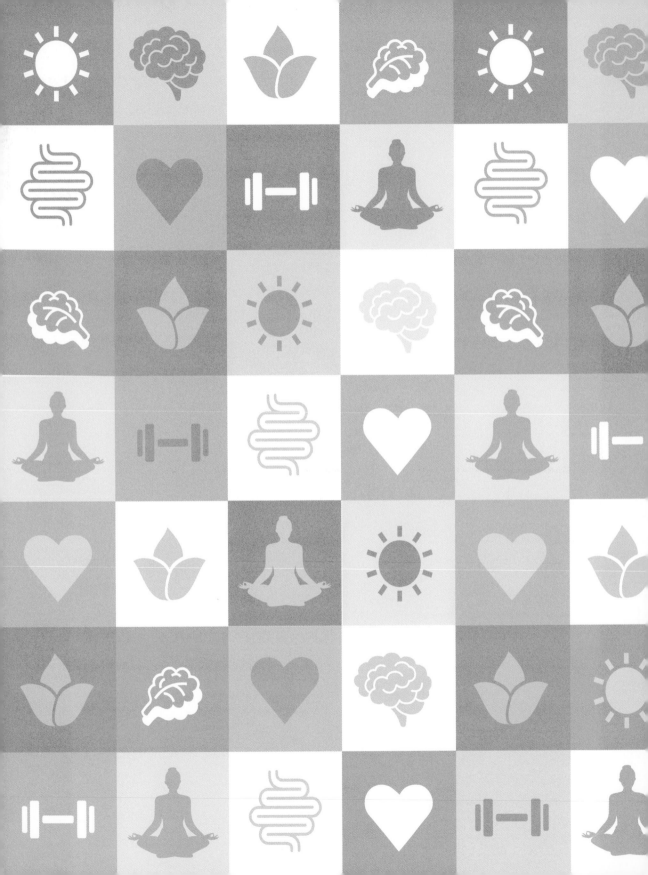

chapter 15

ALL THE RECIPES . . .

I'm a lover of food.
So much so that I went to the French
Culinary Institute here in New York
City in my mid-twenties to learn how to
become a real expert in the kitchen.

My program was a Classic French Cooking + Farm to Table Immersion program, and this earthly element connected me to healthy farming practices, eating local and seasonal, and cooking for flavor and nutrition.

I'm always looking for ways to make traditional comfort food more anti-inflammatory and better for the body. Given how many alternatives are now available (everything from healthier oils to gluten alternatives) there's no reason why you need to sacrifice taste and flavor for health. The truth is, you *can* eat healthy and have the food be delicious.

As you know, the Love Wellness Plan is not about deprivation. It's about learning how to eat amazing food that swaps out inflammatory ingredients for ones that are gentler on your gut and body, and your brain and vagina by extension. I love getting especially creative with dairy-free sauces and dressings and replacing gluten with alternatives that are just as satisfying and comforting.

The following recipes represent my go-to meals. They're all gluten-free, and the majority don't require dairy products. You'll remember that some cheese (like goat or sheep's milk) is allowed in the Plan, and you'll notice I've included it here and there. Most of these recipes serve one to four people, so increase the ingredients as necessary if you're cooking for a family or bigger group! And don't be afraid to play around with the ingredient amounts when it comes to herbs and oils. The amounts of ingredients I've included are all approximate, as everyone has their own preferences. (Just don't triple the amount of goat cheese *every* time!)

I've organized these recipes into groups like breakfast, lunch, and dinner, but feel free to pick and choose based on what your body is telling you. I love a salad for breakfast as an example and have included one in the breakfast section of the recipes. Whether you need a full meal or a quick and delicious snack, there's something in here for every time of the day. Some recipes look more like complete meals and others are great as sides that can be mixed and matched. Be creative, feel free to make tweaks, and enjoy how delicious anti-inflammatory eating for your GBV-axis harmony can be.

Following are twenty-four of my favorite recipes that make cooking well—and eating well—as easy and delicious as possible. I've tried to make sure that each recipe (except for sauces, dressings, sides, and desserts) can be a complete meal if you want it to be. You can mix and match recipes for multiple course meals, too.

Enjoy!

MICROBIOME SUPPORT SMOOTHIE

MAKES 1 SMOOTHIE

PREP: 5 minutes

BLEND TIME: 1 minute

The Microbiome Support Smoothie is my go-to daily breakfast (or lunch, or snack) that gets you all the nutrients your body needs while being anti-inflammatory and great for your gut. It contains protein, fiber, and nutritious fats, *and* it is dairy-free and gluten-free. I prefer using a protein powder that combines beef protein and chicken egg protein (Paleo Pro is a great brand). Chocolate is my favorite flavor, but feel free to go with vanilla or something else you like. Fun tip for those who use Love Wellness products: You can even add your Sparkle Fiber or Daily Love supplements directly to this smoothie by opening up your supplement capsules into the powder!

1 serving of the chocolate protein powder (at least 20 grams of protein)

¼ cup crushed ice (optional; if you like your smoothie really cold)

8 ounces water or preferred nut milk

2 tablespoons raw almond butter

½ cup of organic spinach

Daily supplements (with capsules opened and contents added to smoothie if you prefer to incorporate them into this drink rather than swallowing the supplements with water)

IN a blender mix the protein powder with ice, water or nut milk, almond butter, and spinach.

IF you prefer to add your supplements to the smoothie, break open the capsules and add the contents to the mix.

BLEND together for 30 seconds to 1 minute.

ENJOY!

GHEE BREAKFAST EGGS

SERVES 1

PREP: 5 minutes

COOK TIME: 5 minutes

This healthy breakfast is one of my favorites. Tastes amazing and combines good fats, protein, and fiber? Yes, please. If you don't know about it, ghee is sometimes described as a low-dairy version of butter as the milk solids have been removed from the final product. Eggs cooked slowly with ghee are out-of-this-world-delicious—nutty, creamy, and totally filling.

2 tablespoons ghee

2 organic, pasture-raised eggs

Salt and pepper to taste

½ avocado, thinly sliced

1 handful of organic pea shoots, sunflower sprouts, or similar

Hot sauce to taste

IN a nonstick pan melt the ghee over low heat. Crack open the eggs into a bowl and whisk together while the ghee melts. When melted, add the eggs to the pan and, using a spatula, slowly scramble them until they are soft and fluffy. Keep the heat low the entire time you are cooking, and add salt and pepper at the end to taste.

PLATE the eggs with avocado, topped with organic pea shoots or your sprout of choice.

ADD a tablespoon or two of hot sauce on the side for a little extra heat and flavor.

CAULIFLOWER BREAKFAST BOWL

SERVES 1

PREP: 10 minutes

COOK TIME: 15 minutes

This is a favorite breakfast of mine that packs lots of flavor with the yummy crunch of well-cooked sausage. Cauliflower rice is an excellent base that contains fiber and good carbohydrates, and it easily absorbs the flavor of the garlic and chorizo while cooking. The texture you can achieve with cauliflower rice makes it an especially satisfying meal that feels and tastes like comfort food.

2 tablespoons avocado oil

2 cloves garlic, minced

2 ounces of crumbly pork chorizo or other crumbly sausage (like turkey)

1 cup frozen organic cauliflower rice

Salt and pepper to taste

3 tablespoons organic parsley leaves, roughly chopped

1 organic, pasture-raised egg

¼ avocado, sliced

ADD 1 tablespoon of avocado oil to a nonstick pan. On medium heat, quickly sauté the garlic (about 30 seconds is fine).

CRUMBLE your sausage of choice into the pan and cook until it begins to get brown and crunchy. Remove from the pan and set aside.

IN the same pan, add the cauliflower rice and cook together until the cauliflower is soft and tender, about 7 to 10 minutes. Add the sausage back to the pan once the cauliflower is ready. Season with salt and pepper.

REMOVE from heat and stir in parsley leaves. Set aside in a serving bowl.

IN a separate nonstick pan, fry the egg with the remaining tablespoon of avocado oil over medium heat. Season with salt and pepper.

TOP the cauliflower sausage base with the fried egg and avocado slices and dig in.

BREAKFAST SALAD

SERVES 1–2

PREP: 5 minutes

COOK TIME: 5 minutes

Call me crazy but I love having a salad for breakfast. Hear me out: It's tough to find a light and delicious breakfast, let alone a savory one. My body craves vegetables in the morning for some reason, and this filling breakfast salad gives me the energy I need to get through my mornings. As a bonus, the quinoa and goat cheese make the meal feel savory, without being at all heavy. Try it. Once you're on the breakfast salad train, you won't want to get off.

2 cups organic arugula

⅔ cup cooked quinoa

1 ounce crumbled goat cheese

½ cup chopped pistachios and almonds (mixed)

1 handful of organic blueberries

Drizzle of olive oil (about 1 tablespoon) and balsamic vinegar (about 2 teaspoons)

Salt and pepper to taste

IN a bowl combine the arugula, cooked quinoa, goat cheese, nuts, and blueberries.

DRIZZLE with the olive oil and balsamic vinegar. Salt and pepper to taste.

GOAT CHEESE EGG CUPS

MAKES 12 EGG CUPS

PREP: 20 minutes

COOK TIME: 25–30 minutes

I'm a huge fan of egg cups because you can make a bunch over the weekend and have them for the rest of the week as a perfect grab-and-go breakfast. They also work as a midday snack! I've given you one of my favorite variations of an egg cup that's herbacious and creamy, but you could swap out my ingredients for any vegetable, add hot sauce, or whatever floats your boat.

1 teaspoon avocado oil

¾ cup sage sausage, crumbled

4 ounces goat cheese, crumbled

12 small eggs

Salt and pepper to taste

1½ tablespoons organic sage, chopped (either fresh or dried is fine)

1½ tablespoons organic rosemary, chopped (either fresh or dried is fine)

1 muffin/cupcake tin

12 paper/silicone muffin/cupcake baking cups

PREHEAT oven to 350°F and place 12 muffin baking cups in the muffin tin.

IN a medium pan, heat the avocado oil and brown the sage sausage. I like the Farmer John version but you can always cook plain pork sausage and add dried sage to the mix.

SPOON the sausage and goat cheese (about a tablespoon of each) into each muffin cup.

CRACK an egg into each cup, covering the sausage and goat cheese.

TOP with salt, pepper, and a sprinkle of sage and rosemary.

BAKE for 25–30 minutes or until the eggs are firm.

RANCH REPLACEMENT DRESSING

MAKES 2 CUPS

PREP: 5 minutes

This beloved Ranch Replacement Dressing is my brilliant mom Ellen's recipe. She came up with this ranch alternative (that's more delicious and sophisticated than the classic—and dairy/gluten-free) that pairs perfectly with any salad, and even works as a great dipping sauce for a bowl of turkey meatballs and roasted veggies. It will thicken up a bit in the fridge, but it is a thinner dressing than what you expect from traditional ranch. We like it this way, but if you prefer a thicker dressing, just add a bit more mayo and seasoning.

1 cup avocado mayo (my fave is from Primal Kitchen)

1 cup unsweetened almond milk (MALK is my favorite for this)

1 tablespoon red wine vinegar

1 tablespoon lemon juice

1 heaping teaspoon each: dried tarragon, dried parsley, dried dill, garlic powder, onion powder

1 teaspoon salt

1 teaspoon pepper

ADD the wet ingredients to blender or bowl.

ADD the dry ingredients to the wet ingredients.

MIX by blending or by whisking together.

POUR the contents into a squeeze bottle and refrigerate. It's good for about 7–10 days, and the flavor will intensify over time—just make sure to shake before using!

GREEN TANG DRESSING

MAKES 2 CUPS

PREP: 10 minutes

Do you love green goddess dressing? Here's my flavorful version called Green Tang. It's delicious with just about anything, and trust me, don't skip the anchovies. They add a great umami flavor to this, no fishy taste at all. You'll thank me later! Green Tang Dressing is perfect with your roasted vegetables or a fried egg, or to dip your quesadillas into.

¼ cup fresh mint

¼ cup fresh dill

¼ cup fresh tarragon

¼ cup fresh basil

¼ cup fresh cilantro

¼ cup fresh parsley

Big squeeze of lemon

2–3 tablespoons olive oil

2 cloves garlic

4 anchovies (the ones in oil)

1 cup avocado mayo

½ teaspoon salt

1 teaspoon pepper

WASH and remove the stems from the herbs. Pat the herbs dry, and put them into a blender with the lemon juice and olive oil.

BLEND until smooth (if too thick, add an extra splash of olive oil or water).

ADD garlic, anchovies, and avocado mayo, and blend until smooth.

SEASON with salt and pepper.

POUR the contents into a squeeze bottle or other airtight container and store in the refrigerator. This will last about 7–10 days!

CHORIZO AND GOAT CHEESE QUESADILLAS

SERVES 4–6

PREP: 10 minutes

COOK TIME: 30 minutes

Did you know you can eat quesadillas on an anti-inflammatory diet? Okay, okay, I promise this isn't a joke. My sister's Chorizo and Goat Cheese Quesadilla recipe fits the bill perfectly: It tastes like a treat and follows all the dietary rules of the plan. I love serving these while watching football with my family.

1 tablespoon avocado oil

2 cloves garlic, chopped

½ onion, chopped (about 4 ounces)

Half a package of pork chorizo sausage (the kind that crumbles, about 5–6 ounces)

12 gluten-free tortillas

8 ounces goat cheese

Large handful of chopped organic parsley, stems removed

Salt and pepper to taste

PREHEAT the oven to 400°F. In a medium pan heat the avocado oil. Add the chopped garlic and cook for 1 minute over medium heat before adding the chopped onion. Cook for another minute, then add the chorizo to the pan.

BROWN these ingredients together until some of the chorizo has a nice crunch to it.

LAY 6 of the tortillas onto a baking sheet covered in parchment paper. Press your preferred amount of goat cheese onto each tortilla.

ADD a nice spoonful of the chorizo, onion, and garlic to each tortilla, about 2 tablespoons per tortilla.

SPRINKLE with parsley leaves and add a second tortilla to the top of each mixture.

SPRAY the top and bottom of the quesadilla with a small misting of avocado oil and cook in the oven for about 10 minutes, or until the cheese is melted and the tortilla begins to brown.

CUT into pieces and serve.

CRISPY RICE WITH SALMON AND AVOCADO

SERVES 3–4

PREP: 30 minutes

COOK TIME: 60 minutes

Never had crispy rice with salmon, avocado, cucumber, and jalapeños? Prepare to have your mind (and tastebuds) blown. I started making this recipe in late 2021 when I got my first air fryer, and it's been a staple in my house ever since. It's a healthy twist on Crispy Rice with Spicy Tuna (a popular dish in many Japanese restaurants). If you can find raw sushi-grade salmon go for that. If you can't, regular salmon you cook in a pan is fine. I'll give you both variations of the recipe.

1 cup short-grain white rice

2 tablespoons rice wine vinegar

½ to 1 teaspoon salt (adjust to taste)

1–2 teaspoons sugar

1 tablespoon avocado oil (if cooking salmon)

½ pound raw sushi-grade salmon (keep raw) **OR** ¾ pound regular raw salmon (to cook)

1 tablespoon kewpie mayo

2 tablespoon sriracha

1 tablespoon sesame oil

1 tablespoon soy sauce

1 lime, juiced (about 2 tablespoons)

PREPARE the rice by rinsing it under cold water for at least 10 minutes. I rinse the rice out with fresh water at least once a minute, letting the water fill the bowl, giving the rice a swish with my fingers, then draining and filling again. The goal here is to remove the starch from the outside of each grain so that the rice becomes sticky while cooking. Once your rice can sit in a bowl of water and the water stays mostly clear, it's ready to cook.

COOK the rice according to the package instructions.

IN a small pan, gently heat up the vinegar with salt and sugar until both have dissolved into the vinegar.

POUR the vinegar mixture over the cooked rice and fluff with a fork. Set aside in a bowl.

AT this point, you'll want to heat your air fryer to 400°F (or your regular oven) to preheat.

2 tablespoons of scallions (about 3 scallions)

Cucumber, thinly sliced

1 avocado, smashed

1 jalapeño, finely sliced

Pinch of black sesame seeds

IF you have raw sushi-grade salmon, chop it into very small pieces and place into a bowl in the refrigerator. If you have regular salmon, it's time to quickly sauté it on the stove.

TAKE the salmon filet and season with salt and pepper. Add the avocado oil to a medium pan on medium heat. Place the filet in the pan skin-side up and cook on medium heat until the raw of the meat is almost gone, about 4–5 minutes.

AT this point, flip the filet and turn off the heat, allowing the salmon to finish cooking from the residual heat in the pan. Once done, remove the salmon from its skin using a fork or sharp knife and place the cooked fish into a bowl, flaking it into small pieces.

NOW you'll have either raw or cooked salmon in a bowl. Mix together the kewpie mayo, sriracha, sesame oil, soy sauce, lime juice, and scallions in a bowl. Slowly add to the salmon and gently mix together until you achieve desired taste and consistency. If you want a spicier salmon, add more sriracha. If you're hoping for a bit more robust flavor, add a few more drops of soy sauce. Place the salmon back into the fridge.

NOW it's time to form the crispy rice patties. Prepare the air fryer pan with a piece of parchment paper sprayed with cooking oil (avocado).

USING a small ice cream scoop dipped in water, fill the scoop with sticky rice and press onto the parchment paper, flattening a bit until it forms a disk. Continue until all the rice is formed into disks.

SPRAY the top of the rice with avocado oil and place into the air fryer. Each air fryer is different so you'll need to watch the rice closely to determine when to flip the patties. I cook mine for about 10 minutes before I flip, then finish with another 5–7 minutes until the rice is a light golden-brown color and crunchy.

WHEN cooked, remove the rice from the oven and top each disk with 1 tablespoon of the salmon mixture. If you have leftover salmon, put it back in the fridge and enjoy it the next day on its own.

ONCE each disk has been graced with a delicious spoonful of salmon, top each one with a slice of cucumber, avocado, and jalapeño.

SPRINKLE with black sesame seeds and enjoy.

BROCCOLI AND BACON QUICHE

MAKES 2 QUICHES

PREP: 15 minutes

COOK TIME: 45 minutes

I grew up on quiche. It's so delightful. Full of protein, good carbs from veggies, and a taste that is very comforting. I like this version with a gluten-free crust swapped in because it makes it accessible for more people with dietary restrictions and it's perfect for this plan. Quiche works for breakfast, lunch, dinner, or a snack. Here's a classic recipe for you to enjoy.

8 pieces crispy bacon (about ½ cup per quiche)

2 cups chopped organic broccoli

15 medium organic free-range eggs

½ cup almond milk, unsweetened

1 teaspoon salt

1 teaspoon pepper

2 gluten-free pie crusts (I find them in the freezer aisle)

PREHEAT the oven to 375°F on the convection bake setting.

FRY the bacon in a pan and chop the broccoli into bite-sized pieces.

THEN whisk the eggs in a medium-sized bowl, stir in almond milk, and add a healthy pinch of salt and pepper.

POKE small holes all over the raw pie crust, then layer the broccoli and the bacon into the crusts.

POUR the egg mixture over the broccoli and bacon.

BAKE at the convection setting for 30–35 minutes, until the egg mixture is firm.

BROCCOLI PASTA SALAD

SERVES 6–8

PREP: 30 minutes

COOK TIME: 2–3 hours (including time to chill)

Who doesn't love pasta salad? To make it anti-inflammatory and perfect for your microbiome, I've made this version both gluten- and dairy-free by using gluten-free pasta and my mom's Ranch Replacement Dressing. This is perfect for a weekend snack or backyard barbecue and is delicious once it's had about an hour or two for the flavors to combine in the refrigerator.

1 cup Ranch Replacement Dressing

8–10 pieces bacon

Head of organic broccoli, chopped

15–20 cherry tomatoes

1 large organic cucumber, chopped

1 organic red pepper, chopped

1 box gluten free pasta

Salt, pepper, and lemon to taste

FIRST, make the Ranch Replacement Dressing (see page 201) and store in the refrigerator.

COOK the bacon in a sauté pan until crunchy and let cool, then crumble into pieces.

CHOP all the veggies into bite-sized pieces and set aside.

COOK the pasta in a large pot of water that has been well-seasoned with salt. You want the pasta water to taste salty like the sea before you add pasta so that it's well seasoned when cooked.

WHEN the pasta is cooked to al dente, place it in a colander and immediately rinse with cold water. Then place the pasta in a bowl.

COMBINE the pasta, bacon, and veggies, and slowly start adding the dressing until the pasta and veggies are well-coated (or dressed to your liking).

ADD salt, pepper, and a squeeze of lemon to taste.

COOL in the fridge for 1 hour and then enjoy.

CLASSIC MEATBALLS

YIELDS ABOUT 15 MEATBALLS

PREP: 15 minutes

COOK TIME: 20 minutes

I'm a huge fan of meatballs. They're incredibly versatile and not just for pairing with pasta. I often eat them with a big bowl of arugula and oven-roasted vegetables, topped with my mom's Ranch Replacement Dressing. You can enjoy them with any side you like, and this recipe makes enough for one or two people to have enough for about three days.

1 pound meat (I like to combine pork and beef, but turkey or lamb is great, too)

2 organic free-range eggs

1 tablespoon chopped organic garlic

¼ cup finely diced white onion

Handful organic parsley, about ¼ cup chopped

½ teaspoon red pepper flakes

Handful of gluten-free breadcrumbs

Salt and pepper to taste

2 tablespoons olive oil

IN a mixing bowl combine all the ingredients except the olive oil.

HEAT a large sauté pan on the stove and add a small amount of olive oil. Take a very small piece of the meatball mixture and flatten into a disk in the pan. When flattened, it should brown up in about 1 minute per side. If it's seasoned well, turn off the heat and form the meatballs into even, round balls on a piece of parchment paper. If the tester needs more seasoning, add more salt and pepper and do your taste test again. This small step will ensure the meatballs are perfectly seasoned.

WHEN you're satisfied with the flavor and once you've formed the meatballs with your hands or a spoon, you're ready to cook. Turn the pan back on to medium heat and add more olive oil if necessary. Add all the meatballs to the pan, and turn to the other side after about 5 minutes, once the first side is browned.

BROWN all sides of the meatballs and enjoy with zoodles or a salad.

SPATCHCOCK CHICKEN

SERVES 3–4

PREP: 15 minutes

COOK TIME: 45–60 minutes

Spatchcocking a chicken is the easiest way to roast a chicken that is juicy and full of flavor. The method can be intimidating at first—trust me, I felt the same way—but once you've made this dish, you'll never want to roast a chicken the normal way again. I even spatchcock my turkey on Thanksgiving because it cooks evenly and browns so well. If you need a visual guide, look at a video on YouTube for how to perform this technique.

1 organic chicken

1 tablespoon salt

1 tablespoon pepper

Chopped fresh herbs like organic rosemary, sage, and thyme (about 2 tablespoons of each)

3 tablespoons olive oil

PREHEAT the oven to 450°F. Rinse and dry the chicken completely by patting with paper towels. If there is a giblet bag, remove and discard.

HERE'S where it gets tricky, but you can do this. Place the chicken breast-side down on a cutting board. With a very sharp pair of kitchen scissors, starting at the neck opening, cut down one side of the spine, then the other. Cut across at the base, and then remove the spine.

ON a sheet pan covered with parchment paper, flatten the chicken by opening the bird up and placing the interior side on the sheet pan (skin should be up, facing you).

SEASON the whole bird (the inside, too). You're going to want to spread the olive oil all over your bird quickly because the salt application will start to form beads of water on the skin and prevent good browning. I like to combine a mixture of kosher salt, pepper, and my chopped herbs for easy seasoning into a small bowl so I don't contaminate everything in my kitchen with chicken hands.

ROAST the chicken for 45 minutes or until done (some ovens may take a bit longer—up to an hour). It's done when the internal temperature is 165°F.

REMOVE the chicken from the oven and let sit for 5–10 minutes before carving.

CLASSIC CRUNCHY TACOS

SERVES 3–4

PREP: 30 minutes

COOK TIME: 30 minutes

I t's impossible for me to go a week without having some variation of this recipe. My mom used to make it all the time for us as kids, and it's one of those recipes that is so good that my friends never believe it's healthy. But while this anti-inflammatory meal feels like a cheat day, it's free of both dairy and gluten.

1+ cups avocado oil (1 tablespoon for the meat and 1 cup for frying taco shells)

1 pound ground organic turkey or beef

1 package of Siete Taco Seasoning (about ⅓ cup seasoning per package)

12 medium-sized corn tortillas

Shredded organic lettuce

Shredded organic purple cabbage

1 avocado, sliced or chopped, however you like

Pico de gallo or salsa

IN a large sauté pan, heat 1 tablespoon of avocado oil and cook the ground turkey or beef, breaking the pieces into bite-sized crumbles.

WHEN the pink of the meat is almost gone, add the taco seasoning to the meat and finish browning. If you want the meat to have a nice sauce, add ¼ cup of water to the pan and stir for another minute or two.

SET the temperature to low on the meat or remove from the heat altogether while you make the crispy taco shells.

IN a small frying pan, add 1 cup of avocado oil. Turn the heat on medium-high and heat until you can drop in a sample piece of tortilla and it starts to quickly bubble and fry. Be very careful when you do this to avoid splashing the oil onto your skin. A splash guard can be helpful here.

ONCE the oil is hot, you will fry the tortillas one at a time into the shape of a taco shell. I like using a wooden fork or tongs to help with this. Start by dipping half of the tortilla into the oil, letting it bubble and start to brown. When it starts to brown, flip the uncooked half into the oil while holding the cooked half up out of the oil with fork or tongs. Use your tools to help you shape the tortilla into a taco shape while you fry. If the oil starts to smoke, move the pan off the heat immediately until it cools down. It not, you can find yourself in a kitchen fire situation.

ONCE the tortilla is browned on both sides, place a rolled piece of paper towel in between the shell (where the meat would go if you were making a taco) and set sideways in a large bowl to let the remaining oil drip off into the paper towels.

ONCE the shells are all fried, it's time to assemble the tacos. In each shell put meat, lettuce, cabbage, and avocado and finish with pico de gallo or salsa.

CLASSIC GREEN SOUP

SERVES 4–6

PREP: 30 minutes

COOK TIME: 60 minutes

This fresh and filling green vegetable soup is the genius creation of my friend Kate, a star in the kitchen. She is constantly creating new recipes, and this bright green soup is the perfect go-to when you feel like your body needs a reset or detox. Her Brooklyn kitchen is a constant source of inspiration for me. Kate knows that when it comes to this soup, the brighter the flavor and color, the better!

2–3 celery stalks chopped (about 3 ounces)

2–4 medium-sized garlic cloves depending on preference

1 large leek (soaked to remove dirt, about 8 ounces)

Pinch of chili flakes, optional

1 tablespoon fresh thyme leaves

1–2 dried bay leaves

1–2 zucchini (about 12 ounces total)

1 bunch of broccoli (about 6 ounces once cut into florets)

1 bunch of asparagus (about 10 ounces trimmed and chopped into 1-inch pieces)

6 cups salt-free chicken stock

SAUTÉ the celery, garlic, and leek over medium heat. Add thyme and bay leaves—and a pinch of chili flakes, if you want some heat!

ADD all the vegetables except the spinach and peas and add the stock along with the cashews.

COOK until the veggies are tender and soft, about 20–25 minutes. Remove from heat.

ADD the spinach, half of the peas, and the parsley. Cook using the residual heat until the spinach is barely wilted and still bright green.

REMOVE the bay leaf in preparation for blending together. I like to use a hand-held immersion blender, but Kate uses her Vitamix and ladles it in (if you go this way, just be careful—the soup will be hot).

BLEND until super smooth. If you cooked the spinach just right, the soup should maintain a beautiful bright green color. If the soup seems really thick (like smoothie texture), add additional stock to thin.

Handful of chopped cashews (about 8 whole cashews)

1–2 bunches of spinach (or a 10 ounce box of baby spinach, washed)

5 ounces frozen peas, divided in half (half for the blended soup, and half that will be added at the end for texture)

1 large bunch organic parsley, stems removed

Olive oil, salt, pepper to taste (don't be shy—I use at least 2 teaspoons of kosher salt)

1½ tablespoons lemon juice

SEASON with salt, pepper, and the lemon juice and add in the remaining frozen peas, which will quickly soften in the hot soup.

SERVE drizzled with a bit of olive oil and a parsley leaf garnish.

WHITE BEAN TURKEY CHILI

SERVES 4–6

PREP: 20 minutes

COOK TIME: 3–4 hours

My mom's White Bean Turkey Chili is a chili cook-off winning recipe in our neighborhood. It's a bright-tasting alternative to red and black bean chili, perfect for a cozy night in. What I love about this one is that it's hearty while still tasting light, *and* it's easy to make. Oh, and one batch lasts for days. I use her original recipe without any major tweaks. After all, it's an award winner!

1 teaspoon oregano

1½ teaspoon cumin

½ teaspoon cayenne pepper

1 tablespoon salt

½ teaspoon pepper

2 tablespoons avocado oil

1 pound ground turkey

1 yellow onion

2 cans white beans (cannellini)

1 can diced green chiles, drained

1 cup low-sodium chicken broth

1 bunch green onions

IN a small bowl, combine all the spices, salt, and pepper. Put half of the seasoning in a separate bowl to the side.

IN a large sauté pan, heat up 2 tablespoons of avocado oil. Season the turkey and onion with half of the spice mixture and brown in the pan until the turkey is no longer pink and the onion is translucent, about 10 minutes.

IN a slow-cooker, combine the cooked turkey mixture, white beans, green chiles, chicken broth, and remaining seasoning and cook on low for 3–4 hours.

ONCE the chili has cooked, spoon into bowls and garnish with slices of green onion.

HEALTHY GINGER RAMEN

SERVES 1–2

PREP: 30 minutes

COOK TIME: 20 minutes

I made this Healthy Ginger Ramen years ago on my Instagram, and I still get direct messages asking me for the recipe. I love the flavor combination of ginger and garlic. Don't fear the fish sauce—it gives this soup a depth of flavor you can't achieve without it. The best part is that there is no right or wrong way to make this. Add ingredients and swap stocks to your liking.

2 teaspoons freshly grated ginger

3 cloves minced organic garlic

2 tablespoons olive oil

Handful of organic green onion, chopped and divided for garnish

1 tablespoon chili garlic sauce

Handful shiitake mushrooms (stemmed and sliced)

2 tablespoons fish sauce

3 tablespoons tamari

2 cups chicken stock

2 cups beef stock

2 organic free-range eggs

1–2 packages of angel-hair style Miracle Noodles (1 package per serving)

2 handfuls organic spinach (about 3 ounces)

Handful shredded organic carrots (2 small carrots, about 1 ounce each)

TAKE the freshly grated ginger and minced garlic and add to a pot with the olive oil. Stir together with the chopped green onions and chili sauce. Heat all together over medium heat until lightly browned, about 2 minutes.

ADD the shiitake mushrooms, fish sauce, and tamari to the pot and cook for another minute.

ADD the chicken stock and beef stock to your pot. Let simmer on low.

IN another pot, soft-boil 2 eggs for 6 minutes in boiling water until they are jammy. If you prefer a firmer yolk, boil the eggs for 8 minutes. Then place them in a bowl with cold water and ice, so the eggs are totally submerged, to stop the cooking process.

COOK the noodles according to package directions. Add to the broth.

ADD a handful of spinach and let wilt.

MAKE the bowl! Top the noodles with the carrots, green onion, and soft-boiled eggs. Feel free to add optional toppings like toasted sesame seeds.

CITRUS SALAD

SERVES 4–5

PREP: 45 minutes

This bright salad is a favorite of mine that also combines two of my favorite foods: blood oranges and olives. It's perfect for your winter table, and if you can access citrus fruit year-round, it's a perfect salad to bring to a summer BBQ or pool party. Definitely a crowd-pleaser.

2 large blood oranges (a regular orange works, too), supremed (see the recipe instructions)

1 small grapefruit, supremed

4 cups organic arugula

4 ounces goat cheese, crumbled

2 ounces roasted pistachios

8 ounces Castelvetrano olives, cut into halves

Olive oil, salt, pepper to taste

SUPREME the oranges and grapefruit so that the spongy white tissue (pith) and seeds are removed. This involves using a paring knife to remove both ends of the peel first so you get an orange with a flat top and bottom, then cut the remaining peel while the citrus lies on one of the flesh-exposed flat sides. Once the peel is removed, cut into the pith and remove each piece of flesh, freeing it from the pith and seeds. Feel free to watch a video on YouTube for a visual on how to do this.

ON a platter (I prefer a platter to a bowl for this salad), lay out the arugula followed by the goat cheese, pistachios, and halved olives. Gently place the orange and grapefruit slices onto the salad until evenly distributed.

ADD a pinch of salt and pepper, then drizzle the salad evenly with olive oil before enjoying.

RAW VEGGIE CHOP SALAD

SERVES 6–8

PREP: 30 minutes

COOK TIME: 10–15 minutes

If you watch me cook on my social media channels, you know my Raw Veggie Chop Salad. It is so good, so filling, and easy to make in big batches. I like to chop all my veggies for the week on Sunday, which means I get to have this delicious salad for the rest of the week. It comes together quickly once everything is prepared, and it's a great way to get a huge amount of fiber, fat, and protein in a single meal. It even includes my favorite: gluten-free chicken nuggets chopped into bite-sized pieces.

12 ounces organic broccoli, chopped into bite-sized pieces (about 2–3 ounces per salad)

3 large organic bell peppers in the color of your choice, chopped (about 1 ounce per salad)

Bunch of organic radish, chopped (about 12 radishes)

6 medium organic carrots, chopped

6 mini organic cucumbers, quartered lengthwise and chopped

1 bunch of organic green onions, chopped (about ½ cup)

Handful of organic lettuce

½ avocado (per salad)

4–6 gluten-free chicken nuggets (or protein of your choice)

Handful of roasted sunflower seeds

2 tablespoons Ranch Replacement Dressing

CHOP all the vegetables into bite-sized pieces and store in individual airtight containers.

HEAT up the air fryer or oven and cook the gluten-free chicken nuggets for 10–15 minutes until brown. If you want a protein other than my beloved nuggets, go for it! Once cooked, chop into bite-sized pieces.

TO make one salad, take a handful of the broccoli, a head of lettuce, chopped, and a few tablespoons of the peppers, radishes, carrots, cucumbers, and green onions, and combine in a large bowl.

ADD the nuggets to the veggies along with half an avocado and the sunflower seeds, and toss with 2 tablespoons of Ranch Replacement Dressing.

ENJOY the best raw vegetable salad you've ever had.

RICE WITH PEAS, HERBS, AND FETA

SERVES 4

PREP: 15 minutes

COOK TIME: About 30 minutes

This rice dish is directly inspired by the baked rice dishes of chef Yotam Ottolenghi. I first learned about this masterpiece in his *Simple* cookbook and have been making different variations of it ever since. This version is made with green peas, herbs, and feta cheese, and to make it easier I skip the baking part of the recipe (but definitely look up his baked rice dishes if you want to go the extra mile). The baking he does involves cooking the rice and water in a dish in the oven together with ingredients like butter or olive oil. The result is a brown and crunchy dish, but it can be tricky to get it just right unless you have more advanced kitchen skills. Making rice in a stove-top pan is easier and while not as rich as the original that inspired it, it's still delicious.

1 cup uncooked rice (any long grain is fine)

2 ounces frozen green peas

½ cup chopped organic parsley leaves, fresh mint leaves combined

4 ounces crumbled feta cheese

¼ cup olive oil to coat

1 tablespoon lemon juice

Salt and pepper to taste

COOK up to 1 cup of rice following the directions on the package.

WHEN the rice is still hot, stir in the frozen peas and fresh mint and parsley leaves.

ONCE combined add the feta cheese, olive oil, and lemon juice and stir again.

SEASON with a bit of salt and pepper, and eat while hot!

CREAMY MASHED CAULIFLOWER

SERVES 3–4

PREP: 15 minutes

COOK TIME: 20 minutes

On its own, cauliflower is a brilliant vegetable that easily transforms into tortillas and pizza crusts. My favorite twist on this vegetable is mashed cauliflower. It's a lower-carb substitute to mashed potatoes that's perfect with any weeknight meal. Cauliflower is creamy on its own, so it doesn't need much to taste delightful . . . but the broth and ghee definitely get it there.

1 head organic cauliflower

2 garlic cloves, minced

1 small leek, soaked and rinsed to remove dirt, and then minced

2 tablespoons ghee

1 cup chicken broth

Salt and pepper to taste

WASH and cut the cauliflower into small florets. Put them into a microwave-safe bowl, add a few tablespoons of water, cover and steam in the microwave for 3–4 minutes until the florets are tender. I prefer this method to boiling the cauliflower just to save time.

SAUTÉ the minced garlic and leeks in 1 tablespoon of ghee over low heat until both are soft and slightly browned (about 5–10 minutes).

MEANWHILE, boil the chicken broth in a pan at medium heat and set aside.

ADD the cauliflower, garlic, and leeks to a food processor along with 2–3 tablespoons of boiling chicken broth.

PULSE until the vegetables lose their shape and start to come together in a creamier consistency. Add more chicken broth, in small amounts, until you achieve your desired consistency.

POUR the mash into a bowl and season with salt and pepper.

TOP with another tablespoon of ghee and serve.

ROASTED VEGETABLE PLATTER

SERVES 4

PREP: 30 minutes

COOK TIME: 25–35 minutes

If you're like me, you add roasted vegetables to your plate whenever you get the chance. I eat them on their own, with a side of Ranch Replacement Dressing, paired with meatballs, mixed in with arugula for an earthy salad, and more. The possibilities are endless. The best part? A tray of roasted vegetables is one of the easiest and tastiest dishes to pull off.

2 cups butternut squash, cut into 1 inch pieces

1 cup carrots, cut into 1 inch pieces

Or, an optional additional variety of vegetables like parsnips and potatoes cut into 1 inch pieces

1 large onion, cut into large slices

Olive oil to coat

Salt and pepper to taste

Handful of dried herbs like parsley, oregano, and thyme

PREHEAT the oven to 400°F.

WASH and dry the vegetables and cut into equal-sized 1-inch pieces so that they are more likely to cook evenly.

IN a bowl, coat the chopped vegetables with olive oil, salt, pepper, and your dried herbs.

LAY the veggies onto a sheet pan covered with parchment paper, spreading them out evenly.

ROAST the veggies for about 25–35 minutes. Remove the pan from the oven halfway through and give them a toss so the pieces brown evenly.

ENJOY on their own or as a side.

CHOCOLATE CUPCAKES

MAKES ABOUT 18 CUPCAKES

PREP: 20 minutes

COOK TIME: 30 to 40 minutes

My mom makes a cake version of this that is topped with whipped cream. Don't get me wrong, I love a good cake—but perfectly rich and decadent cupcakes? Yes, please. These single-serving cupcakes are made with cassava flour, which is my new favorite flour for gluten-free baking.

2 cups cassava flour

1 cup pure cocoa powder

1½ cups King Arthur's Baking Sugar Alternative

1½ teaspoon baking powder

1½ teaspoon baking soda

1 teaspoon vanilla extract

1 cup almond milk, unsweetened

1 cup water

2 organic free-range eggs

½ cup olive oil

FOR THE TOPPING

1 can of chilled coconut cream, with most liquid poured off

Raspberries

PREHEAT the oven to 350°F. In a medium-sized bowl, mix all the dry ingredients.

IN another bowl, mix all the wet ingredients.

POUR the wet into the dry ingredients and whisk until the batter is smooth and well-combined.

POUR the batter into a well-greased and lined cupcake tray and bake at 350°F for 30 to 40 minutes.

FINISH with a topping of your choice (or eat them as is, sort of like a brownie). If you want to make whipped cream using a can of coconut cream you'll get a nice dairy-free topping that pairs well with raspberries.

TO make the coconut whipped cream I recommend chilling a can of coconut cream in the refrigerator overnight. Pour off and reserve the clear liquid in the can and whip the almost-solid coconut cream in a chilled metal bowl until soft peaks form. If you want it to be a bit airier, add a tiny bit of the reserved liquid when whipping.

SWEET POTATO BROWNIES

SERVES 8

PREP: 15 minutes:

COOK TIME: 1–2 hours

This recipe is so simple to make, and an absolute favorite of mine. This "brownie" can be cut up into tiny squares or slices and it retains tons of moisture because of the sweet potato base. I like to add chocolate chips for some extra flavor but you could skip them if you aren't a chocolate fan. It doesn't rise at all, so expect the final product to be a slightly gooey but thick and delicious "brownie" that is about an inch in height.

1–2 sweet potatoes

1 organic free-range egg

⅓ cup melted coconut oil

1 cup cassava flour

⅓ cup King Arthur's Baking Sugar Alternative

1 teaspoon salt

⅓ cup dark chocolate chips

PREHEAT the oven to 400°F.

STICK 1–2 sweet potatoes with a fork a few times so they don't explode in the oven, and roast for 45–60 minutes.

LOWER the oven to 375°F.

PEEL the skin from the sweet potatoes, using a kitchen towel to protect your hands from the heat, and discard the skin. Mash the sweet potatoes until smooth.

MIX wet ingredients (eggs, melted coconut oil, sweet potatoes) together in one bowl.

MIX the dry ingredients (cassava flour, sugar, and salt) together in another bowl.

COMBINE the wet ingredients with the dry ones.

FOLD in the chocolate chips.

GREASE a bread pan (a 1-pound loaf pan works), pour in mixture, and bake for 45 minutes.

ACKNOWLEDGMENTS

First and foremost, this book would not be possible without the support of my incredible family. When I first began Love Wellness, my family members were my most ardent supporters. I was going through a challenging moment in my life, and I'm so thankful that I have unshakeable support from my mom, dad, brother, sister, their partners and children. Their willingness to have open conversations about our bodies gave me the confidence needed to focus on the personal care category and share my own story.

The idea for a book really came from the Love Wellness team. We are always looking for ways to share my story, and after years of social media videos, marketing emails, and speaking engagements, putting pen to paper in the form of a book was the logical next step. I'm so thankful that I have the support of such a great team. At the time this manuscript is due, that includes Joanne, Killips, Aaly, Katrina, Jessica, Amanda, Anna, Anna, Kacey, Madeline, Olivia, Erica, Jon, Rene, Temi, Madi, Lexi, Drew, Lainee, Alicia, Chandler, Abby, Kelsey, Martine, Lindsay, Caroline, Isabel, and James. I'm sure more have joined us by the time of publication—thank you. Also, thank you to Kate, Robert, and Megan at Encore for being such wonderful guides on this journey together.

Thank you to Valerie Frankel for not only being delightful, but also brilliant. Your time and dedication to this project will forever be appreciated. You helped me find my voice, define my perspective, and share my story.

Thank you to the entire Aardvark/Ultra Literary team, especially Peter McGuigan who helps us soar and Kathy Huck who keeps us focused.

Thanks to Casey Barber for her excellent recipe testing.

At Dey Street, I couldn't be more appreciative of Carrie Thornton. You were the first to share our vision and understand the impact we could have with this project. You are a champion for women everywhere. And thank you to my editor, Anna Montague. Your commentary when editing our recipe section always brings a smile to my face.

A huge thank-you to Joanne Gray, Amanda Russo, and the entire Goodwin team. You jump in and save the day, always.

Finally, a special thanks to my medical advisors, personal doctors, nutritionists, and friends. Janine Higbie is a talented Certified Dietitian Nutritionist responsible for the bulk of the Love Wellness Plan and is one of the most considerate, thoughtful people I know. She cares deeply about her clients (which now include all of you reading this book). Thank you to Dr. Jodie Horton, Dr. Shweta Desai, Dr. Gabrielle Francis, Dr. Michael Breus, and Dr. Irwin Grosman. Your teachings are invaluable.

NOTES

INTRODUCTION

1. USDA, Agricultural Research Service, 2019. "Usual Nutrient Intake from Food and Beverages, by Gender and Age, What We Eat in America," NHANES 2013–2016.

CHAPTER 1: EMPOWERED SELF-ADVOCACY

1. American Psychiatric Association. Diagnostic and statistical manual of mental disorders. 2nd ed. pg 39–41. American Psychiatric Association; Washington, D.C., USA: 1968.

2. Fairweather, D., Rose, N.R. Women and autoimmune diseases. *Emerg Infect Dis*. 2004 Nov;10(11):2005–11. doi: 10.3201/eid1011.040367. PMID: 15550215; PMCID: PMC3328995.

3. Maas, A.H., Appelman, Y.E. Gender differences in coronary heart disease. *Neth Heart J*. 2010; 18(12):598–602. doi:10.1007/s12471–010–0841–y.

4. https://www.gao.gov/assets/gao-01-286r.pdf.

5. Nowogrodzki, A. Inequality in medicine. *Nature*, 550, S18–S19 (2017). https://doi.org/10.1038/550S18a.

6. Liu, K.A., Mager, N.A. Women's involvement in clinical trials: historical perspective and future implications. *Pharm Pract (Granada)*. 2016;14(1):708. doi:10.18549/PharmPract.2016.01.708.

7. Chen, E.H., Shofer, F.S., Dean, A.J., Hollander, J.E., Baxt, W.G., Robey, J.L., Sease, K.L., Mills, A.M. Gender disparity in analgesic treatment of emergency department patients with acute abdominal pain. *Acad Emerg Med*. 2008 May;15(5):414–8. doi: 10.1111/j.1553–2712.2008.00100.x. PMID: 18439195.

CHAPTER 2: LEAKY GUT

1. Lagkouvardos, I., Overmann, J., Clavel, T. Cultured microbes represent a substantial fraction of the human and mouse gut microbiota. *Gut Microbes*. 2017 Sep 3;8(5):493–503. doi: 10.1080/19490976.2017.1320468. Epub 2017 Apr 18. PMID: 28418756; PMCID: PMC5628658.

2. Moeller, A.H., Caro-Quintero, A., Mjungu, D., Georgiev, A.V., Lonsdorf, E.V., Muller, M.N., Pusey, A.E., Peeters, M., Hahn, B.H., Ochman, H. Cospeciation of gut microbiota with hominids. *Science*. 2016 Jul 22;353(6297):380–2. doi: 10.1126/science.aaf3951. PMID: 27463672; PMCID: PMC4995445.

3. Feltman, Rachel. "You can earn $13,000 a year selling your poop." *The Washington Post*. January 29, 2015.

4. Ciorba, M.A. A gastroenterologist's guide to probiotics. *Clin Gastroenterol and Hepatol*. 2012;10(9):960–968. doi:10.1016/j.cgh.2012.03.024.

5. Tulstrup, M.V., Christensen, E.G., Carvalho, V., et al. Antibiotic Treatment Affects Intestinal Permeability and Gut Microbial Composition in Wistar Rats Dependent on Antibiotic Class. *PLoS One*. 2015;10(12):e0144854. Published 2015 Dec 21. doi:10.1371/journal.pone.0144854.

6. Bjarnason, I., Takeuchi, K. Intestinal permeability in the pathogenesis of NSAID-induced enteropathy. *J Gastroenterol*. 2009;44 Suppl 19:23–9. doi: 10.1007/s00535–008–2266–6. Epub 2009 Jan 16. PMID: 19148789.

7. Konturek, P.C., Brzozowski, T., Konturek, S.J. Stress and the gut: pathophysiology, clinical consequences, diagnostic approach and treatment options. *J Physiol Pharmacol*. 2011 Dec;62(6):591–9. PMID: 22314561.

8. Binienda, A., Twardowska, A., Makaro, A., Salaga, M. Dietary carbohydrates and lipids in the pathogenesis of leaky gut syndrome: An overview. *Int J Mol Sci*. 2020;21(21):8368. Published 2020 Nov 8. doi:10.3390/ijms21218368.

9. Wu, H.J., Wu, E. The role of gut microbiota in immune homeostasis and autoimmunity. *Gut Microbes*. 2012;3(1):4–14. doi:10.4161/gmic.19320.

10. Drago, S., El Asmar, R., Di Pierro, M., Grazia Clemente, M., Tripathi, A., Sapone, A., Thakar, M., Iacono, G., Carroccio, A., D'Agate, C., Not, T., Zampini, L., Catassi, C., Fasano, A. Gliadin, zonulin and gut permeability: Effects on celiac and non-celiac intestinal mucosa and intestinal cell lines. *Scand J Gastroenterol*. 2006 Apr; 41(4):408–19. doi: 10.1080/00365520500235334. PMID: 16635908.

11. Fasano, A. Zonulin, regulation of tight junctions, and autoimmune diseases. *Ann N Y Acad Sci*. 2012;1258(1):25–33. doi:10.1111/j.1749-6632.2012.06538.x.

CHAPTER 3: LEAKY BRAIN

1. Obrenovich, M.E.M. Leaky Gut, Leaky Brain? *Microorganisms*. 2018;6(4):107. Published 2018 Oct 18. doi:10.3390/microorganisms6040107.

2. Braniste, V., Al-Asmakh, M., Kowal, C., Anuar, F., Abbaspour, A., Tóth, M., Korecka, A., Bakocevic, N., Ng, L.G., Kundu, P., Gulyás, B., Halldin, C., Hultenby, K., Nilsson, H., Hebert, H., Volpe, B.T., Diamond, B., Pettersson, S. The gut microbiota influences blood-brain barrier permeability in mice. *Sci Transl Med*. 2014 Nov 19;6(263):263ra158. doi: 10.1126/scitranslmed.3009759. Erratum in: *Sci Transl Med*. 2014 Dec 10;6(266):266er7. Guan, Ng Lai [corrected to Ng, Lai Guan]. PMID: 25411471; PMCID: PMC4396848.

3. Logsdon, A.F., Erickson, M.A., Rhea, E.M., Salameh, T.S., Banks, W.A. Gut reactions: How the blood-brain barrier connects the microbiome and the brain. *Exp Biol Med (Maywood)*. 2018 Jan;243(2):159–165. doi: 10.1177/1535370217743766. Epub 2017 Nov 23. PMID: 29169241; PMCID: PMC5788145.

4. Sharon, G., Sampson, T.R., Geschwind, D.H., Mazmanian, S.K. The central nervous system and the gut microbiome. *Cell*. 2016;167(4):915–932. doi:10.1016/j.cell.2016.10.027

5. Arzani, M., Jahromi, S.R., Ghorbani, Z. et al. Gut-brain axis and migraine headache: A comprehensive review. *J Headache Pain* 21, 15 (2020). https://doi.org/10.1186/s10194-020-1078-9.

6. Benedict, C., Vogel, H., Jonas, W., et al. Gut microbiota and glucometabolic alterations in response to recurrent partial sleep deprivation in normal-weight young individuals. *Mol Metab*. 2016;5(12):1175–1186. Published 2016 Oct 24. doi:10.1016/j.molmet.2016.10.003.

7. Gundry, Stephen R. *The Energy Paradox: What to Do When Your Get-Up-and-Go Has Got Up and Gone*. Pg. 98. Harper Wave, 2021.

8. Smith, R.P., Easson, C., Lyle, S.M., Kapoor, R., Donnelly, C.P., Davidson, E.J., et al. (2019) Gut microbiome diversity is associated with sleep physiology in humans. *PLoS ONE* 14(10): e0222394. https://doi.org/10.1371/journal.pone.0222394.

9. Hurtado-Alvarado, G., Domínguez-Salazar, E., Pavon, L., Velázquez-Moctezuma, J., Gómez-González, B. Blood-brain barrier disruption induced by chronic sleep loss: Low-grade inflammation may be the link. *J Immunol Res*. 2016;2016:4576012. doi:10.1155/2016/4576012.

10. Sarkar, A., Lehto, S.M., Harty, S., Dinan, T.G., Cryan, J.F., Burnet, P.W.J. Psychobiotics and the manipulation of bacteria-gut-brain signals. *Trends Neurosci*. 2016;39(11):763–781. doi:10.1016/j.tins.2016.09.002.

11. Benton, D., Williams, C., Brown, A. Impact of consuming a milk drink containing a probiotic on mood and cognition. *Eur J Clin Nutr*. 2007 Mar;61(3):355–61. doi: 10.1038/sj.ejcn.1602546. Epub 2006 Dec 6. PMID: 17151594.

12. Messaoudi, M., Lalonde, R., Violle, N., Javelot, H., Desor, D., Nejdi, A., Bisson, J.F., Rougeot, C., Pichelin, M., Cazaubiel, M., Cazaubiel, J.M. Assessment of psychotropic-like properties of a probiotic formulation (*Lactobacillus helveticus* R0052 and *Bifidobacterium longum* R0175) in rats and human subjects. *Br J Nutr*. 2011 Mar;105(5):755–64. doi: 10.1017/S0007114510004319. Epub 2010 Oct 26. PMID: 20974015.

13. Steenbergen, L., Sellaro, R., van Hemert, S., Bosch, J.A., Colzato, L.S. A randomized controlled trial to test the effect of multispecies probiotics on cognitive reactivity to sad mood. *Brain Behav Immun*. 2015 Aug;48:258–64. doi: 10.1016/j.bbi.2015.04.003. Epub 2015 Apr 7. PMID: 25862297.

14. Fasano, A. Zonulin, regulation of tight junctions, and autoimmune diseases. *Ann N Y Acad Sci*. 2012;1258(1):25–33. doi:10.1111/j.1749-6632.2012.06538.x.

CHAPTER 4: LEAKY VAGINA

1. Waters, C.M., Bassler, B.L. Quorum sensing: Cell-to-cell communication in bacteria. *Annu Rev Cell Dev Biol*. 2005;21:319–46. doi: 10.1146/annurev.cellbio.21.012704.131001. PMID: 16212498.

2. Dobson, A., Cotter, P.D., Ross, R.P., Hill, C. Bacteriocin production: A probiotic trait? *Appl Environ Microbiol*. 2012 Jan;78(1):1–6. doi: 10.1128/AEM.05576–11. Epub 2011 Oct 28. PMID: 22038602; PMCID: PMC3255625.

3. Crann, S.E., Cunningham, S., Albert, A., Money, D.M., O'Doherty, K.C. Vaginal health and hygiene practices and product use in Canada: A national cross-sectional survey. *BMC Womens Health*. 2018 Mar 23;18(1):52. doi: 10.1186/s12905-018-0543-y. PMID: 29566756; PMCID: PMC5865287.

4. Ananthapadmanabhan, K.P., Lips, A., Vincent, C., Meyer, F., Caso, S., Johnson, A., Subramanyan, K., Vethamuthu, M., Rattinger, G., Moore, D.J. pH-induced alterations in stratum corneum properties. *Int J Cosmet Sci*. 2003 Jun;25(3):103–12. doi: 10.1046/j.1467-2494.2003.00176.x. PMID: 18494892.

5. Kim, T.S., Kim, C.Y., Lee, H.K., Kang, I.H., Kim, M.G., Jung, K.K., Kwon, Y.K., Nam, H.S., Hong, S.K., Kim, H.S., Yoon, H.J., Rhee, G.S. Estrogenic activity of persistent organic pollutants and parabens based on the stably transfected human estrogen receptor-a transcriptional activation assay (OECD TG 455). *Toxicol Res*. 2011 27(3):181–4.

6. Brown, J.M., Hess, K.L., Brown, S., Murphy, C., Waldman, A.L., Hezareh, M. Intravaginal practices and risk of bacterial vaginosis and candidiasis infection among a cohort of women in the United States. *Obstet Gynecol*. 2013 Apr;121(4):773–780. doi: 10.1097/AOG.0b013e31828786f8. PMID: 23635677.

7. Tone, Andrea. *Devices and Desires: A History of Contraception in America*. Hill & Wang Pub, 2001.

8. Eschenbach, D.A., Thwin, S.S, Patton, D.L., Hooton, T.M., Stapleton, A.E., Agnew, K., Winter, C., Meier, A., Stamm, W.E. Influence of the normal menstrual cycle on vaginal tissue, discharge, and microflora. *Clinical Infectious Diseases*, Volume 30, Issue 6, June 2000, Pages 901–907, https://doi.org/10.1086/313818.

9. Al-Badr, A., Al-Shaikh, G. Recurrent urinary tract infections management in women: A review. *Sultan Qaboos Univ Med J*. 2013;13(3):359–367. doi:10.12816/0003256

10. Foxman, B. Epidemiology of urinary tract infections: incidence, morbidity, and economic costs. *Am J Med*. 2002 Jul 8;113 Suppl 1A:5S-13S. doi: 10.1016/s0002-9343(02)01054-9. PMID: 12113866.

11. Renard, J., Ballarini, S., Mascarenhas, T., Zahran, M., Quimper, E., Choucair, J., Iselin, C.E. Recurrent lower urinary tract infections have a detrimental effect on patient quality of life: A

prospective, observational study. *Infect Dis Ther*. 2014 Dec 18;4(1):125–35. doi: 10.1007/s40121–014–0054–6. Epub ahead of print. PMID: 25519161; PMCID: PMC4363217.

12. https://www.niddk.nih.gov/health-information/urologic-diseases/bladder-infection-uti-in-adults/symptoms-causes.

13. Alanazi, M.Q., Alqahtani, F.Y., Aleanizy, F.S. An evaluation of E. coli in urinary tract infection in emergency department at KAMC in Riyadh, Saudi Arabia: retrospective study. *Ann Clin Microbiol Antimicrob*. 2018;17(1):3. Published 2018 Feb 9. doi:10.1186/s12941–018–0255-z.

CHAPTER 5: PATHWAYS

1. Furness, J.B. The enteric nervous system and neurogastroenterology. *Nat Rev Gastroenterol Hepatol*. 2012 Mar 6;9(5):286–94. Doi: 10.1038/nrgastro.2012.32. PMID: 22392290.

2. Pellissier, S., Dantzer, C., Mondillon, L., Trocme, C., Gauchez, A.S., Ducros, V., Mathieu, N., Toussaint, B., Fournier, A., Canini, F., Bonaz, B. Relationship between vagal tone, cortisol, TNF-alpha, epinephrine and negative affects in Crohn's disease and irritable bowel syndrome. *PLoS One*. 2014 Sep 10;9(9):e105328. doi: 10.1371/journal.pone.0105328. PMID: 25207649; PMCID: PMC4160179.

3. Breit, S., Kupferberg, A., Rogler, G., Hasler, G. Vagus nerve as modulator of the brain-gut axis in psychiatric and inflammatory disorders. *Front Psychiatry*. 2018 Mar 13;9:44. doi: 10.3389/fpsyt.2018.00044. PMID: 29593576; PMCID: PMC5859128.

4. Bonaz, B., Bazin, T., Pellissier, S. The vagus nerve at the interface of the microbiota-gut-brain axis. *Front Neurosci*. 2018;12:49. Published 2018 Feb 7. doi:10.3389/fnins.2018.00049.

5. Jungmann, M., Vencatachellum, S., Van Ryckeghem, D., Vögele, C. Effects of cold stimulation on cardiac-vagal activation in healthy participants: Randomized controlled trial. *JMIR Form Res*. 2018;2(2):e10257. Published 2018 Oct 9. doi:10.2196/10257.

6. Kalyani, B.G., Venkatasubramanian, G., Arasappa, R., et al. Neurohemodynamic correlates of 'OM' chanting: A pilot functional magnetic resonance imaging study. *Int J Yoga*. 2011;4(1):3–6. doi:10.4103/0973–6131.78171

7. Vickhoff, B., Malmgren, H., Aström, R., et al. Music structure determines heart rate variability of singers [published correction appears in *Front Psychol*. 2013 Sep 05;4:599]. *Front Psychol*. 2013;4:334. Published 2013 Jul 9. doi:10.3389/fpsyg.2013.00334

8. da Silva, M.A., Dorsher, P.T. Neuroanatomic and clinical correspondences: acupuncture and vagus nerve stimulation. *J Altern Complement Med*. 2014 Apr;20(4):233–40. doi: 10.1089/acm.2012.1022. Epub 2013 Dec 20. PMID: 24359451.

9. He, W., Wang, X., Shi, H., Shang, H., Li, L., Jing, X., Zhu, B. Auricular acupuncture and vagal regulation. *Evid Based Complement Alternat Med*. 2012;2012:786839. doi: 10.1155/2012/786839. Epub 2012 Nov 27. PMID: 23304215; PMCID: PMC3523683.

10. Golec de Zavala, A., Lantos, D., Bowden, D. Yoga poses increase subjective energy and state self-esteem in comparison to 'power poses' [published correction appears in *Front Psychol*. 2018 Feb 09;9:149]. *Front Psychol*. 2017; 8:752. Published 2017 May 11. doi:10.3389/fpsyg.2017.00752.

11. Kok, B.E., Coffey, K.A., Cohn, M.A., Catalino, L.I., Vacharkulksemsuk, T., Algoe, S.B., Brantley, M., Fredrickson, B.L. How positive emotions build physical health: perceived positive social connections account for the upward spiral between positive emotions and vagal tone. *Psychol Sci*. 2013 Jul 1;24(7):1123–32. doi: 10.1177/0956797612470827. Epub 2013 May 6. Erratum in: Psychol Sci. 2016 Jun;27(6):931. PMID: 23649562.

12. Ohinata, K., Takemoto, M., Kawanago, M., Fushimi, S., Shirakawa, H., Goto, T., Asakawa, A., Komai, M. Orally administered zinc increases food intake via vagal stimulation in rats. *J Nutr*. 2009 Mar;139(3):611–6. doi: 10.3945/jn.108.096370. Epub 2009 Jan 21. PMID: 19158231.

13. Bravo, J.A., Forsythe, P., Chew, M.V., Escaravage, E., Savignac, H.M., Dinan, T.G., Bienenstock, J., Cryan, J.F. Ingestion of lactobacillus strain regulates emotional behavior and central GABA receptor expression in a mouse via the vagus nerve. *Proc Natl Acad Sci U S A*. 2011 Sep 20;108(38):16050–5. doi: 10.1073/pnas.1102999108. Epub 2011 Aug 29. PMID: 21876150; PMCID: PMC3179073.

14. Komisaruk, B.R., Whipple, B., Crawford, A., Liu, W.C., Kalnin, A., Mosier, K. Brain activation during vaginocervical self-stimulation and orgasm in women with complete spinal cord injury: fMRI evidence of mediation by the vagus nerves. *Brain Res*. 2004 Oct 22;1024(1–2):77–88. doi: 10.1016/j.brainres.2004.07.029. PMID: 15451368.

15. Mantis, N., Rol, N. & Corthésy, B. Secretory IgA's complex roles in immunity and mucosal homeostasis in the gut. *Mucosal Immunol* 4, 603–611 (2011). https://doi.org/10.1038/mi.2011.41

16. Costa, R.J.S., Snipe, R.M.J., Kitic, C.M., Gibson, P.R. Systematic review: Exercise-induced gastrointestinal syndrome-implications for health and intestinal disease. *Aliment Pharmacol Ther*. 2017 Aug;46(3):246–265. doi: 10.1111/apt.14157. Epub 2017 Jun 7. PMID: 28589631.

17. Caldara, M., Friedlander, R.S., Kavanaugh, N.L., Aizenberg, J., Foster, K.R., Ribbeck, K. Mucin biopolymers prevent bacterial aggregation by retaining cells in the free-swimming state. *Curr Biol*. 2012 Dec 18;22(24):2325–30. doi: 10.1016/j.cub.2012.10.028. Epub 2012 Nov 8. PMID: 23142047; PMCID: PMC3703787.

18. Bergstrom, K., Shan, X., Casero, D., Batushansky, A., Lagishetty, V., Jacobs, J.P., Hoover, C., Kondo, Y., Shao, B., Gao, L., Zandberg, W., Noyovitz, B., McDaniel, J.M., Gibson, D.L., Pakpour, S., Kazemian, N., McGee, S., Houchen, C.W., Rao, C.V., Griffin, T.M., Sonnenburg, J.L., McEver, R.P., Braun, J., Xia, L. Proximal colon-derived O-glycosylated mucus encapsulates and modulates the microbiota. *Science*. 2020 Oct 23;370(6515):467–472. doi: 10.1126/science.aay7367. PMID: 33093110; PMCID: PMC8132455.

19. Birchenough, G., Schroeder, B.O., Bäckhed, F., Hansson, G.C. Dietary destabilisation of the balance between the microbiota and the colonic mucus barrier. *Gut Microbes*. 2019;10(2):246–250. doi:10.1080/19490976.2018.1513765.

20. Monin, L., Whettlock, E.M., Male, V. Immune responses in the human female reproductive tract. *Immunology*. 2020 Jun;160(2):106–115. doi: 10.1111/imm.13136. Epub 2019 Nov 11. PMID: 31630394; PMCID: PMC7218661.

21. Kavanaugh, N.L., Zhang, A.Q., Nobile, C.J., Johnson, A.D., Ribbeck, K. Mucins suppress virulence traits of Candida albicans. *mBio*. 2014 Nov 11;5(6):e01911. doi: 10.1128/mBio.01911–14. PMID: 25389175; PMCID: PMC4235211.

22. O'Connell, C.M., Ferone, M.E. *Chlamydia trachomatis* Genital Infections. *Microb Cell*. 2016 Sep 5;3(9):390–403. doi: 10.15698/mic2016.09.525. PMID: 28357377; PMCID: PMC5354567.

23. Orange, J.S. Human natural killer cell deficiencies and susceptibility to infection. *Microbes Infect*. 2002 Dec;4(15):1545–58. doi: 10.1016/s1286-4579(02)00038–2. PMID: 12505527.

24. Spinner, M.A., Sanchez, L.A., Hsu, A.P., Shaw, P.A., Zerbe, C.S., Calvo, K.R., Arthur, D.C., Gu, W., Gould, C.M., Brewer, C.C., Cowen, E.W., Freeman, A.F., Olivier, K.N., Uzel, G., Zelazny, A.M., Daub, J.R., Spalding, C.D., Claypool, R.J., Giri, N.K., Alter, B.P., Mace, E.M., Orange, J.S., Cuellar-Rodriguez, J., Hickstein, D.D., Holland, S.M. GATA2 deficiency: A protean disorder of hematopoiesis, lymphatics, and immunity. *Blood*. 2014 Feb 6;123(6):809–21. doi: 10.1182/blood-2013-07-515528. Epub 2013 Nov 13. PMID: 24227816; PMCID: PMC3916876.

25. Martyn, F., McAuliffe, F.M., Wingfield, M. The role of the cervix in fertility: Is it time for a reappraisal? *Hum Reprod*. 2014 Oct 10;29(10):2092–8. doi: 10.1093/humrep/deu195. Epub 2014 Jul 27. PMID: 25069501.

26. Wira, C.R., Rodriguez-Garcia, M., Patel, M.V. The role of sex hormones in immune protection of the female reproductive tract. *Nat Rev Immunol*. 2015 Apr;15(4):217–30. doi: 10.1038/nri3819. Epub 2015 Mar 6. PMID: 25743222; PMCID: PMC4716657.

27. Kutteh, W.H., Moldoveanu, Z., Mestecky, J. Mucosal immunity in the female reproductive tract: Correlation of immunoglobulins, cytokines, and reproductive hormones in human cervical mucus around the time of ovulation. *AIDS Res Hum Retroviruses*. 1998 Apr;14 Suppl 1:S51–5. PMID: 9581884.

28. Gaskins, A.J., Chavarro, J.E. Diet and fertility: A review. *Am J Obstet Gynecol*. 2018;218(4):379–389. doi:10.1016/j.ajog.2017.08.010.

29. Lach, G., Schellekens, H., Dinan, T.G., Cryan, J.F. Anxiety, depression, and the microbiome: A role for gut peptides. *Neurotherapeutics*. 2018 Jan;15(1):36–59. doi: 10.1007/s13311–017–0585–0. PMID: 29134359; PMCID: PMC5794698.

30. Yano, J.M., Yu, K., Donaldson, G.P., et al. Indigenous bacteria from the gut microbiota regulate host serotonin biosynthesis. [Published correction appears in *Cell*. 2015 Sep 24;163:258.] *Cell*. 2015;161(2):264–276. doi:10.1016/j.cell.2015.02.047.

31. Mazzoli, R., Pessione, E. The neuro-endocrinological role of microbial glutamate and GABA signaling. *Front Microbiol*. 2016;7:1934. Published 2016 Nov 30. doi:10.3389/fmicb.2016.01934.

32. Desbonnet, L., Garrett, L., Clarke, G., Kiely, B., Cryan, J.F., Dinan, T.G. Effects of the probiotic Bifidobacterium infantis in the maternal separation model of depression. *Neuroscience*. 2010 Nov 10;170(4):1179–88. doi: 10.1016/j.neuroscience.2010.08.005. Epub 2010 Aug 6. PMID: 20696216.

33. Bravo, J.A., Forsythe, P., Chew, M.V., Escaravage, E., Savignac, H.M., Dinan, T.G., Bienenstock, J., Cryan, J.F. *Proceedings of the National Academy of Sciences* Sep 2011, 108 (38) 16050–16055; doi: 10.1073/pnas.1102999108.

34. Schmidt, K., Cowen, P.J., Harmer, C.J., Tzortzis, G., Errington, S., Burnet, P.W. Prebiotic intake reduces the waking cortisol response and alters emotional bias in healthy volunteers. *Psychopharmacology (Berl)*. 2015;232(10):1793–1801. doi:10.1007/s00213–014–3810–0.

35. Clarke, G., Stilling, R.M., Kennedy, P.J., Stanton, C., Cryan, J.F., Dinan, T.G.. Minireview: Gut microbiota: The neglected endocrine organ. *Mol Endocrinol*. 2014 Aug;28(8):1221–38. doi: 10.1210/me.2014–1108. Epub 2014 Jun 3. PMID: 24892638; PMCID: PMC5414803.

36. Lyte, M. (2013) Microbial endocrinology in the microbiome-gut-brain axis: How bacterial production and utilization of neurochemicals influence behavior. *PLoS Pathog* 9(11): e1003726. https://doi.org/10.1371/journal.ppat.1003726.

37. Steenbergen, L., et al. A randomized controlled trial to test the effect of multi-species probiotics on cognitive reactivity to sad mood. *Brain, Behavior, and Immunity* 48 (2015): 258–64. https://doi.org/10.1016/j.bbi.2015.04.003.

38. Valles-Colomer, M., et al. The neuroactive potential of the human gut micro-biota in quality of life and depression. *Nature Microbiology* 4, no. 4 (2019): 623–32. https://doi.org/10.1038/s41564–018–0337-x.

39. Amabebe, E., Anumba, D.O.C. Psychosocial Stress, Cortisol Levels, and Maintenance of Vaginal Health. *Front Endocrinol (Lausanne)*. 2018;9:568. Published 2018 Sep 24. doi:10.3389/fendo.2018.00568.

40. Coria-Avila, G.A., Herrera-Covarrubias, D., Ismail, N., Pfaus, J.G. The role of orgasm in the development and shaping of partner preferences. *Socioaffect Neurosci Psychol*. 2016;6:31815. Published 2016 Oct 25. doi:10.3402/snp.v6.31815.

CHAPTER 6: HAPPY GUT

1. Imhann, F., Bonder, M.J., Vich Vila, A., Fu, J., Mujagic, Z., Vork, L., Tigchelaar, E.F., Jankipersadsing, S.A., Cenit, M.C., Harmsen, H.J., Dijkstra, G., Franke, L., Xavier, R.J., Jonkers, D., Wijmenga, C., Weersma, R.K., Zhernakova, A. Proton pump inhibitors affect the gut microbiome. *Gut*. 2016 May;65(5):740–8. doi: 10.1136/gutjnl-2015-310376. Epub 2015 Dec 9. PMID: 26657899; PMCID: PMC4853569.

2. Jalanka, J., Major, G., Murray, K., et al. The effect of psyllium husk on intestinal microbiota in constipated patients and healthy controls. *Int J Mol Sci*. 2019;20(2):433. Published 2019 Jan 20. doi:10.3390/ijms20020433.

3. Kajla, P., Sharma, A., Sood, D.R. Flaxseed—a potential functional food source. *J Food Sci Technol*. 2015 Apr;52(4):1857–71. doi: 10.1007/s13197-014-1293-y. Epub 2014 Feb 28. PMID: 25829567; PMCID: PMC4375225.

4. Licht, T.R., Hansen, M., Bergström, A., Poulsen, M., Krath, B.N., Markowski, J., Dragsted, L.O., Wilcks, A. Effects of apples and specific apple components on the cecal environment of conventional rats: role of apple pectin. *BMC Microbiol*. 2010 Jan 20;10:13. doi: 10.1186/1471-2180-10-13. PMID: 20089145; PMCID: PMC2822772.

5. Slavin, J. Fiber and prebiotics: Mechanisms and health benefits. *Nutrients*. 2013;5(4):1417–1435. Published 2013 Apr 22. doi:10.3390/nu5041417.

6. Patterson, M.A., Maiya, M., Stewart, M.L. Resistant starch content in foods commonly consumed in the United States: A narrative review. *J Acad Nutr Diet*. 2020 Feb;120(2):230–244. doi: 10.1016/j.jand.2019.10.019. PMID: 32040399.

7. Sorrenti, V., Ali, S., Mancin, L., Davinelli, S., Paoli, A., Scapagnini, G. Cocoa polyphenols and gut microbiota interplay: Bioavailability, prebiotic effect, and impact on human health. *Nutrients*. 2020;12(7):1908. Published 2020 Jun 27. doi:10.3390/nu12071908.

8. Wirngo, F.E., Lambert, M.N., Jeppesen, P.B. The physiological effects of dandelion (*Taraxacum Officinale*) in Type 2 Diabetes. *Rev Diabet Stud*. 2016;13(2–3):113–131. doi:10.1900/RDS.2016.13.113.

9. Zhang, Ning & Huang, Xuesong & Zeng, Yanhua & Wu, Xiyang & Peng, Xichun. (2013). Study on prebiotic effectiveness of neutral garlic fructan in vitro. *Food Science and Human Wellness*. 2. 10.1016/j.fshw.2013.07.001.

10. Munim, Adil & Rod, Michel & Tavakoli, Hamed & Hosseinian, Farah. (2017). An analysis of the composition, health benefits, and future market potential of the Jerusalem artichoke in Canada. *Journal of Food Research*. 6. 69. 10.5539/jfr.v6n5p69.

11. Valeur, J., Puaschitz, N.G., Midtvedt, T., Berstad, A. Oatmeal porridge: Impact on microflora-associated characteristics in healthy subjects. *Br J Nutr*. 2016 Jan 14;115(1):62–7. doi: 10.1017/S0007114515004213. Epub 2015 Oct 29. PMID: 26511097.

12. Kumar, V.P., Prashanth, K.V.H., Venkatesh, Y.P. Structural analyses and immunomodulatory properties of fructo-oligosaccharides from onion (Allium cepa). *Carbohydr Polym*. 2015 Mar 6;117:115–122. doi: 10.1016/j.carbpol.2014.09.039. Epub 2014 Sep 28. PMID: 25498616.

13. de Oliveira Leite, A.M., Miguel, M.A, Peixoto, R.S., Rosado, A.S., Silva, J.T., Paschoalin, V.M. Microbiological, technological and therapeutic properties of kefir: a natural probiotic beverage. *Braz J Microbiol*. 2013 Oct 30;44(2):341–9. doi: 10.1590/S1517-83822013000200001. PMID: 24294220; PMCID: PMC3833126.

14. Park, K.Y., Jeong, J.K., Lee, Y.E., Daily, J.W. 3rd. Health benefits of kimchi (Korean fermented vegetables) as a probiotic food. *J Med Food*. 2014 Jan;17(1):6–20. doi: 10.1089/jmf.2013.3083. PMID: 24456350.

15. Denter, J., Bisping, B. Formation of B-vitamins by bacteria during the soaking process of soybeans for tempe fermentation. *Int J Food Microbiol*. 1994 Apr;22(1):23–31. doi: 10.1016/0168-1605(94)90004-3. PMID: 8060790.

16. Ríos-Covián, D., Ruas-Madiedo, P., Margolles, A., Gueimonde, M., de Los Reyes-Gavilán, C.G., Salazar, N. Intestinal short chain fatty acids and their link with diet and human health. *Front Microbiol*. 2016;7:185. Published 2016 Feb 17. doi:10.3389/fmicb.2016.00185.

17. Żółkiewicz, J., Marzec, A., Ruszczyński, M., Feleszko, W. Postbiotics—A step beyond pre- and probiotics. *Nutrients*. 2020 Jul 23;12(8):2189. doi: 10.3390/nu12082189. PMID: 32717965; PMCID: PMC7468815.

18. Kotani, Y., Shinkai, S., Okamatsu, H., Toba, M., Ogawa, K., Yoshida, H., Fukaya, T., Fujiwara, Y., Chaves, P.H., Kakumoto, K., Kohda, N. Oral intake of *Lactobacillus pentosus* strain b240 accelerates salivary immunoglobulin A secretion in the elderly: A randomized, placebo-controlled, double-blind trial. *Immun Ageing*. 2010 Aug 26;7:11. doi: 10.1186/1742-4933-7-11. PMID: 20796295; PMCID: PMC2936365.

19. Silva YP, Bernardi A, Frozza RL. The role of short-chain fatty acids from gut microbiota in gut-brain communication. *Front Endocrinol* (Lausanne). 2020;11:25. Published 2020 Jan 31. doi:10.3389/fendo.2020.00025.

20. Caspani G., Kennedy S., Foster J.A., Swann J. Gut microbial metabolites in depression: understanding the biochemical mechanisms. *Microb Cell*. 2019;6(10):451–481. Published 2019 Sep 27. doi:10.15698/mic2019.10.693.

21. Di Sabatino, A., Morera, R., Ciccocioppo, R., Cazzola, P., Gotti, S., Tinozzi, F.P., Tinozzi, S., Corazza, G.R. Oral butyrate for mildly to moderately active Crohn's disease. *Aliment Pharmacol Ther*. 2005 Nov 1;22(9):789–94. doi: 10.1111/j.1365-2036.2005.02639.x. PMID: 16225487.

22. Goswami, C., Iwasaki, Y., Yada, T. Short-chain fatty acids suppress food intake by activating vagal afferent neurons. *J Nutr Biochem*. 2018 Jul;57:130–135. doi: 10.1016/j.jnutbio.2018.03.009. Epub 2018 Mar 17. PMID: 29702431.

23. Cavallari, J.F., Fullerton, M.D., Duggan, B.M., Foley, K.P., Denou, E., Smith, B.K., Desjardins, E.M., Henriksbo, B.D., Kim, K.J., Tuinema, B.R., Stearns, J.C., Prescott, D., Rosenstiel, P., Coombes, B.K., Steinberg, G.R., Schertzer, J.D. Muramyl dipeptide-based postbiotics mitigate obesity-induced insulin resistance via IRF4. *Cell Metab*. 2017 May 2;25(5):1063–1074.e3. doi: 10.1016/j.cmet.2017.03.021. Epub 2017 Apr 20. PMID: 28434881.

24. McAfee, A.J., McSorley, E.M., Cuskelly, G.J., et al. Red meat from animals offered a grass diet increases plasma and platelet n-3 PUFA in healthy consumers. *Br J Nutr*. 2011;105(1):80–89. doi:10.1017/S0007114510003090.

25. Zhang, X., Zou, Q., Zhao, B., Zhang, J., Zhao, W., Li, Y., Liu, R., Liu, X., Liu, Z. Effects of alternate-day fasting, time-restricted fasting and intermittent energy restriction DSS-induced on colitis and behavioral disorders. *Redox Biol*. 2020 May;32:101535. doi: 10.1016/j.redox.2020.101535. Epub 2020 Apr 10. Erratum in: Redox Biol. 2021 Aug;44:101955. PMID: 32305005; PMCID: PMC7162980.

CHAPTER 7: HAPPY BRAIN

1. Cai, D.J., Mednick, S.A., Harrison, E.M., Kanady, J.C., Mednick, S.C. REM, not incubation, improves creativity by priming associative networks. *Proc Natl Acad Sci USA*. 2009 Jun 23;106(25):10130–4. doi: 10.1073/pnas.0900271106. Epub 2009 Jun 8. PMID: 19506253; PMCID: PMC2700890.

2. Besset, A., Tafti, M., Villemin, E., Borderies, P., Billiard, M. Effects of zolpidem on the architecture and cyclical structure of sleep in poor sleepers. *Drugs Exp Clin Res*. 1995;21(4):161–9. PMID: 8529530.

3. Chang, A.-M., Aeschbach, D., Duffy, J.F., Czeisler, C.A. (2014). Evening use of light-emitting eReaders negatively affects sleep, circadian timing, and next-morning alertness. *PNAS*, 112(4), 1232–1237.

4. Daniel, S., Limson, J.L., Dairam, A., Watkins, G.M., Daya, S. Through metal binding, curcumin protects against lead- and cadmium-induced lipid peroxidation in rat brain homogenates and against lead-induced tissue damage in rat brain. *J Inorg Biochem*. 2004 Feb;98(2):266–75. doi: 10.1016/j.jinorgbio.2003.10.014. PMID: 14729307.

5. Małkiewicz, M.A., Szarmach, A., Sabisz, A. et al. Blood-brain barrier permeability and physical exercise. *J Neuroinflammation* 16, 15 (2019). https://doi.org/10.1186/s12974-019-1403-x.

6. van Praag, H. Exercise and the brain: Something to chew on. *Trends Neurosci*. 2009;32(5):283–290. doi:10.1016/j.tins.2008.12.007.

7. von Holstein-Rathlou, S., Petersen, N.C., Nedergaard, M. Voluntary running enhances glymphatic influx in awake behaving, young mice. *Neurosci Lett*. 2018;662:253–258. doi:10.1016/j.neulet.2017.10.035.

8. van Praag, H. Exercise and the brain: Something to chew on. *Trends Neurosci*. 2009;32(5):283–290. doi:10.1016/j.tins.2008.12.007

9. Lee, H., Xie, L., Yu, M., Kang, H., Feng, T., Deane, R., Logan, J., Nedergaard, M., Benveniste, H. The effect of body posture on brain glymphatic transport. *J Neurosci*. 2015 Aug 5;35(31):11034–44. doi: 10.1523/JNEUROSCI.1625–15.2015. PMID: 26245965; PMCID: PMC4524974.

CHAPTER 8: HAPPY VAGINA

1. van Eijk, A.M., Zulaika, G., Lenchner, M., Mason, L., Sivakami, M., Nyothach, E., Unger, H., Laserson, K., Phillips-Howard, P. (2019). Menstrual cup use, leakage, acceptability, safety, and availability: A systematic review and meta-analysis. *The Lancet Public Health*. 4. 10.1016/S2468–2667(19)30111–2.

2. Nonfoux, L., Chiaruzzi, M., Badiou, C., Baude, J., Tristan, A., Thioulouse, J., Muller, D., Prigent-Combaret, C., Lina, G. Impact of currently marketed tampons and menstrual cups on *Staphylococcus aureus* growth and toxic shock syndrome Toxin 1 production *In Vitro*. *Appl Environ Microbiol*. 2018 May 31;84(12):e00351–18. doi: 10.1128/AEM.00351–18. PMID: 29678918; PMCID: PMC5981080.

3. Dfarhud, D., Malmir, M., Khanahmadi, M. Happiness & health: The biological factors—systematic review article. *Iran J Public Health*. 2014;43(11):1468–1477.

4. NCHS, National Survey of Family Growth, 2015–2017.

5. Spinillo, A., Capuzzo, E., Nicola, S., Baltaro, F., Ferrari, A., Monaco, A. The impact of oral contraception on vulvovaginal candidiasis. *Contraception*. 1995 May;51(5):293–7. doi: 10.1016/0010–7824(95)00079-p. PMID: 7628203.

6. Khalili, H., Higuchi, L.M., Ananthakrishnan, A.N., Richter, J.M., Feskanich, D., Fuchs, C.S., Chan, A.T. Oral contraceptives, reproductive factors and risk of inflammatory bowel disease. *Gut*. 2013 Aug;62(8):1153–9. doi: 10.1136/gutjnl-2012–302362. Epub 2012 May 22. PMID: 22619368; PMCID: PMC3465475.

7. Baker, J.M., Al-Nakkash, L., Herbst-Kralovetz, M.M. Estrogen-gut microbiome axis: Physiological and clinical implications. *Maturitas*. 2017 Sep;103:45–53. doi: 10.1016/j.maturitas.2017.06.025. Epub 2017 Jun 23. PMID: 28778332.

8. Vostalova, J., Vidlar, A., Simanek, V., Galandakova, A., Kosina, P., Vacek, J., Vrbkova, J., Zimmermann, B.F., Ulrichova, J., Student, V. Are high proanthocyanidins key to cranberry efficacy in the prevention of recurrent urinary tract infection? *Phytother Res*. 2015 Oct;29(10):1559–67. doi: 10.1002/ptr.5427. Epub 2015 Aug 13. PMID: 26268913.

9. Domenici, L., Monti, M., Bracchi, C., Giorgini, M., Colagiovanni, V., Muzii, L., Benedetti Panici, P. D-mannose: A promising support for acute urinary tract infections in women. A pilot study. *Eur Rev Med Pharmacol Sci*. 2016 Jul;20(13):2920–5. PMID: 27424995.

10. Yang PJ, Pham J, Choo J, Hu DL. Duration of urination does not change with body size. Proc Natl Acad Sci U S A. 2014 Aug 19;111(33):11932-7. doi: 10.1073/pnas.1402289111. Epub 2014 Jun 26. PMID: 24969420; PMCID: PMC4143032.

CHAPTER 9: LEAKS AND PATHWAYS: THE FULL DIGEST

1. Byrd, A.L., Belkaid, Y., Segre, J.A. The human skin microbiome. *Nat Rev Microbiol.* 2018 Mar;16(3):143–155. doi: 10.1038/nrmicro.2017.157. Epub 2018 Jan 15. PMID: 29332945.

2. Nakatsuji, T., Chen, T.H., Butcher, A.M., Trzoss, L.L., Nam, S.J., Shirakawa, K.T., Zhou, W., Oh, J., Otto, M., Fenical, W., Gallo, R.L. A commensal strain of *Staphylococcus epidermidis* protects against skin neoplasia. *Sci Adv.* 2018 Feb 28;4(2):eaao4502. doi: 10.1126/sciadv.aao4502. PMID: 29507878; PMCID: PMC5834004.

3. Bowe, W.P., Logan, A.C. Acne vulgaris, probiotics and the gut-brain-skin axis—back to the future? *Gut Pathog.* 2011 Jan 31;3(1):1. doi: 10.1186/1757-4749-3-1. PMID: 21281494; PMCID: PMC3038963.

4. Selway, C.A., Mills, J.G., Weinstein, P., Skelly, C., Yadav, S., Lowe, A., Breed, M.F., Weyrich, L.S. Transfer of environmental microbes to the skin and respiratory tract of humans after urban green space exposure. *Environ Int.* 2020 Dec;145:106084. doi: 10.1016/j.envint.2020.106084. Epub 2020 Sep 22. PMID: 32977191.

CHAPTER 10: WEEK 1: PREP WEEK

1. Rao, R., Samak, G. Role of glutamine in protection of intestinal epithelial tight junctions. *J Epithel Biol Pharmacol.* 2012 Jan;5(Suppl 1-M7):47–54. doi: 10.2174/1875044301205010047. PMID: 25810794; PMCID: PMC4369670.

2. Jozkowski, K.N., Herbenick, D., Schick, V., Reece, M., Sanders, S.A., Fortenberry, J.D. Women's perceptions about lubricant use and vaginal wetness during sexual activities. *J Sex Med.* 2013 Feb;10(2):484–92. doi: 10.1111/jsm.12022. Epub 2012 Dec 4. PMID: 23211029.

CHAPTER 11: WEEK 2: LESS OF THE BAD STUFF

1. Caio, G., Lungaro, L., Segata, N., et al. Effect of gluten-free diet on gut microbiota composition in patients with celiac disease and non-celiac gluten/wheat sensitivity. *Nutrients.* 2020;12(6):1832. Published 2020 Jun 19. doi:10.3390/nu12061832.

2. Sandro Drago, Ramzi El Asmar, Mariarosaria Di Pierro, Maria Grazia Clemente, Amit Tripathi Anna Sapone, Manjusha Thakar, Giuseppe Iacono, Antonio Carroccio, Cinzia D'Agate, Tarcisio Not, Lucia Zampini, Carlo Catassi & Alessio Fasano Gliadin, zonulin and gut permeability: Effects on celiac and non-celiac intestinal mucosa and intestinal cell lines, *Scandinavian Journal of Gastroenterology,* 41:4, (2006) 408–419, DOI: 10.1080/00365520500235334.

3. Yin, K.J., Xie, D.Y., Zhao, L., et al. Effects of different sweeteners on behavior and neurotransmitters release in mice. *J Food Sci Technol.* 2020;57(1):113–121. doi:10.1007/s13197-019-04036-6

4. Shil, A., Olusanya, O., Ghufoor, Z., Forson, B., Marks, J., Chichger, H. Artificial sweeteners disrupt tight junctions and barrier function in the intestinal epithelium through activation of the sweet taste receptor, T1R3. *Nutrients.* 2020;12(6):1862. Published 2020 Jun 22. doi:10.3390/nu12061862.

5. Bishehsari, F., Magno, E., Swanson, G., et al. Alcohol and gut-derived inflammation. *Alcohol Res.* 2017;38(2):163–171.

CHAPTER 13: WEEK 4: BLISS IS YOURS

1. Simopoulos, A.P. Evolutionary aspects of diet, the omega-6/omega-3 ratio and genetic variation: Nutritional implications for chronic disease. *Biomed Pharmacother.* 2006;60(9):502–507. doi:10.1016/j.biopha.2006.07.080

2. Fetissov, S.O., Laviano, A., Kalra, S., Inui, A. Update on ghrelin. *Int J Pept.* 2010;2010:963501. doi:10.1155/2010/963501.

INDEX

neuroplasticity, 97

neurotransmitters, 89, 126, 174

Nexium, 155

nondominant hand, using, 97

nonstick cookware, 141

NSAIDs, 155

nut flours, 152

nutrient absorption
  difficulties with, xiv
  inner gut wall and, 19

nutrient-dense foods, 56

nutrition
  ongoing balance and, 182–185
  during prep week, 136–140
  during week 2, 150–156
  during week 3, 162–166
  during week 4, 172–175
  see also diet; fiber; recipes

nuts, 165

O

oats, 79, 164

off-gassing, 140

oils, 172–173

omega-3 fatty acids, 52, 61, 83, 84, 95, 105, 138, 172–173, 185

omega-6 fatty acids, 172–173

ongoing balance, 181–189

onions, 79

organic foods/products, 81–84, 86, 123, 137, 139–140, 155–156

orgasms, 69, 111, 119, 125, 144, 157, 167, 176, 186

ovarian cysts, 6

ovaries, 33, 63

ovulation, 60

oxidation, 93–94, 124

oxidative stress, 93–94, 95

oxytocin, 69, 111, 127, 144

P

pads, 104

pancreas, 63

panic attacks, ix–xi

Pap smears, 12

parabens, 38, 81, 103, 142

parasympathetic breathing, 51, 143

parasympathetic nervous system (PNS), 50, 111, 176, 177

parathyroids, 62

pasta, gluten-free, 152

Pasta Salad, Broccoli, 208

patient compliance, 9

peas
  benefits of, 164
  Rice with Peas, Herbs, and Feta, 220

pelvic exams, 12

pelvic floor, 106–108, 125

pelvic nerve, 52

pepsin, 85

perineum, 33, 103

periods, 104–106, 125

personal care cleansers, 37

pesticides, 81

pH levels, in intestinal cavity, 19. *see also* vagina: pH of

phthalates, 38, 81, 103, 142

pineal gland, 62

pituitary gland, 62, 69

plant proteins, 61

plastic, in kitchen, 141

polyethylene glycol (PEG), 37

polyphenols, 162

postbiotics, 77, 80–81

postpartum care, 117, 190

potatoes, 164

prebiotics, 77–79, 138

pregnancy
  discharge during, 41
  mucus and, 61
  nutrition and, 190
  as treatment for hysteria, 4
  UTIs and, 43
  vaginal health and, 116
  see also childbirth

prenatal vitamins, 190

prep week, 135–147

prescription drugs
  blood-brain barrier (BBB) and, 26
  gender differences regarding, 9–10
  sleep and, 91

Prevacid, 155

Prilosec, 75, 155

Proanthocyanidin (Pac), 114

ABOUT THE AUTHOR

Lauren "Lo" Bosworth is the founder and CEO of the total-body-care brand Love Wellness. After experiencing chronic health issues she couldn't fix with traditional drugstore products or prescriptions, she realized there was a need for personal care products driven by body positivity, clean ingredients, and holistic wellness. Since launching the company in 2016, she has expanded Love Wellness to include vaginal health, gut health, and ingestible beauty. Today, she continues to help change the narrative around self-care culture and empower others to feel supported, welcomed, and safe during their wellness journeys.

Bosworth has lived in New York City since 2012 and is from Laguna Beach, California. She is a graduate of UCLA and the French Culinary Institute.